Building Your Family

Building
Your
Family

The Complete Guide
to Donor Conception

Lisa Schuman, LCSW,
and Mark Leondires, MD

ST. MARTIN'S
ESSENTIALS
NEW YORK

First published in the United States by St. Martin's Essentials, an imprint of St. Martin's Publishing Group

BUILDING YOUR FAMILY. Copyright © 2023 by Lisa Schuman and Mark Leondires. All rights reserved. Printed in the United States of America. For information, address St. Martin's Publishing Group, 120 Broadway, New York, NY 10271.

www.stmartins.com

Designed by Steven Seighman

The Library of Congress Cataloging-in-Publication Data is available upon request.

ISBN 978-1-250-86826-8 (hardcover)
ISBN 978-1-250-86827-5 (ebook)

Our books may be purchased in bulk for promotional, educational, or business use. Please contact your local bookseller or the Macmillan Corporate and Premium Sales Department at 1-800-221-7945, extension 5442, or by email at MacmillanSpecialMarkets@macmillan.com.

First Edition: 2023

10 9 8 7 6 5 4 3 2 1

This book is dedicated to Keith, my husband and best friend. This book would not be possible without you. And to our wonderful children, Dylan, Greer, and Julian, connected by our hearts and not our genetics.

—*LS*

This book is dedicated to those who have helped millions bring children into their lives; and to a future where family-building help can be accessible to all. To my husband and children, who have changed me forever, and to three amazing, giving women who brought my family to life.

—*ML*

Contents

Part IV: Preparing for Your Family—
with Gratitude

Building Your Family

Preface

You are reading this book because you are considering building your family through donor conception. Since you are willing to consider donor conception, you can begin to focus on *when* you will be a parent rather than *if* you will. Of course, there are no guarantees, but there are many ways and many resources to build a family. We hope this is one of those resources that empowers you. Help is available, and it can be comforting to know that the majority of people who are open to donor conception are able to have a child.

That is not to minimize the effort it requires and the obstacles you'll face. Building a family through donor conception is not easy or spontaneous. This book will help you know it can work. We know this from extensive firsthand experience, both professional and personal. Family building was a challenging journey for both of us. We want it to be easier for you.

We are confident it will be, not only because you have this book and our decades of experience to guide you, but also because the science continues to advance. Reproductive researchers are constantly coming up with new and better technologies to make the process easier and to increase the odds of successful conception and pregnancy. Improved sperm, egg, and embryo screening, more advanced methods for matching donors with recipients, and better tracking of the use and outcomes of treatment are all smoothing the road that leads to happy families, healthy children, and children with a healthy sense of self. Just as important, the community of donor-conceived children and adults continues to grow, and as it does, we learn more and more about their social-emotional needs and what we can do—starting at the beginning of the process—to help them lead their best lives.

After working with thousands of donors, parents-to-be, and donor-conceived children, we have compiled the information that we believe you are most interested in learning about. In doing so, we hope to save you hours of internet scrolling and sleepless nights not knowing where to find the answers you need, and perhaps even to help you minimize your stress and conflicts with your loved ones. This is the book we wish we'd had when we were building our families. We hope it serves you well.

Introduction

Roberto and Bridget were both successful, busy professionals who were not planning to have children. Then one day, after years of being happy as a two-person family, Bridget realized that she had changed her mind—she wanted to have a baby. She raised the issue with Roberto, and after many talks and much planning, he agreed. Their life together would feel more complete if they had a child to share it with. Unfortunately, by this time, Bridget was thirty-eight, and her eggs were no longer of a high enough quality to create a successful pregnancy. Even after several rounds of fertility treatment, she still wasn't pregnant. That was when she and Roberto decided to use an egg donor.

Lori and Christina were in love, and they badly wanted to share their love with children. They both had grown up with siblings and still maintained close relationships with them. They hoped to have two kids who could develop similar deep bonds, so they came to us for help finding a sperm donor and embarking on their journey. Though they had some misconceptions about the process and many questions, and it was initially difficult for them to agree which of them would carry the first pregnancy, they were committed to learning all they could, as well as to open communication and compromise with each other.

Like Lori and Christina, Benjamin and Brian also wanted children, but complicating matters for them was the fact that Brian's family was very traditional and had never been supportive of their relationship. This was hard for Brian, who didn't know how his parents would react to their decision to have children. On top of that, money was going to be an issue. It would not be easy for Benjamin, a special education teacher, and Brian, a video editor, to pay for the costs associated with using donor eggs and a gestational carrier. Between a loan and some financial assistance from Benjamin's family, they were able to make a feasible plan.

Joanna had been in a serious long-term relationship in her twenties, but in the years after that, her relationships were more casual—not because she was avoiding commitment but because she simply didn't form a deep connection with anyone. She had always wanted to have a child, however, and by the time she was thirty-one, she was seriously considering single parenthood rather than waiting to find the right partner. She joined the online support group Single Mothers by Choice and chatted with several women who had become single parents and others who, like her, were considering it. She also talked with her sister and a close friend, both of whom would be crucial pieces of her support network should she decide to try to conceive with a sperm donor. After weighing all that she'd learned, she decided that she was ready.

All these people eventually became pregnant and had babies using donor conception. All of them had challenges during the process, as everyone does, but they were able to overcome those challenges and build the families they dreamed of because they educated themselves and they had supportive professionals to guide them through the process. Both are necessary. It's our desire to provide you with that education and be your first guide in donor conception. We see hundreds of patients a year, and over the years, we've helped thousands become parents. Every day, patients tell us that they've learned critical information that they hadn't considered, that we spared them from making choices they might later regret, and most important that they feel confident, finally, in embracing donor conception. It truly brings us joy when we help set someone on the right path, when we help them feel understood in their struggle, help them manage the stress of the process, and let them know they are not alone. And of course, nothing brings us more joy than when our patients conceive, get pregnant, and have a child. We often say "we work for baby pictures"! With this book, we will walk you through all you need to know to begin the journey of donor conception and feel confident that you are making the right choices for your future family.

The patients profiled above also had something else that was key: a strong desire to become parents that carried them through the emotional difficulties and the inevitable temporary setbacks. The donor-conception process can be confusing, expensive, time-consuming, and emotionally unsettling. It can be fraught with difficult emotions like shame, loneliness, and hurt. It's not for everyone, and reading this book will help you determine if it's for you. For those who go through the process, their deep yearning to become a parent outweighs the challenges. The reward—finally holding your baby in your arms—we know will make all the work worth it.

If you're considering donor conception, or if you've already decided to pursue it, you know how unfair it feels. If you have infertility, it can feel like your body has let you down while it seems like everyone around you is getting pregnant and having babies. If you are in a same-sex relationship, it can feel like a cruel injustice that you can't simply conceive at home, or even have fertility treatment reimbursed by your insurance carrier like heterosexual couples can. For single parents-to-be, you may wish you had a partner but feel you can't wait any longer to start a family, or you may be determined to do it on your own. Either way, it can feel daunting to face donor conception alone. Like same-sex couples, you may feel insecure, judged, and criticized for your choice by the outside world.

We are here to tell you that it *is* unfair. We wish we could revitalize eggs or create an embryo with two sperm, two eggs, or one sperm or one egg. Science is not there yet, but donor conception is a wonderful option. If you're reading this book, it's likely that you are willing to go to the ends of the earth to build your family. But where do you start? How do you know which questions to ask? As you saw in those patient profiles, people's stories are different. Still, everyone faces the same basic journey and many of the same challenges. For starters, we're guessing that you want advice on how to choose a donor, speak to your future children about their donor origins, and talk about all of this with others. Our book is your guide to navigating your journey from the moment you accept that you need and want to use donor conception. You'll find answers to those questions and many more.

In short, this is your all-in-one guide to not only demystifying an incredibly challenging process—for many, the most difficult process of their lives—but also inspiring confidence that the journey will be a successful one, providing crucial support and encouragement every step of the way.

Who We Are

Together, we have nearly fifty years of experience in donor conception, and we bring professional as well as personal experience.

Lisa

Although I am the happy mother of three children, it wasn't easy getting here. After marriage, I discovered that a medication my mother took while pregnant with me led to a deformity of my uterus. This structural defect caused me to have several miscarriages and years of fertility treatment.

I had always dreamed of being pregnant. I played with

dolls as a child and fantasized about my future family. I used to tell my girlfriends that I couldn't wait to have a huge belly and feel the baby grow inside my body. I had always assumed pregnancy "would just happen" when I wanted it to happen. Why not? This was my plan. It was also my husband Keith's plan. So, after spending my young adult life trying *not* to get pregnant, Keith and I began to try *to* get pregnant. I'll never forget one day when I was pregnant and he said, "I have never been so happy." I felt the same. But it never lasted. Later, watching his heartbreak worsened the pain our infertility was causing me every day.

Eventually, Keith and I did what most desperate people would do—try everything. We tried immunological treatments, drank smelly concoctions from an herbalist in a six-story walk-up in Chinatown, and did acupuncture. I visualized and didn't visualize. I meditated and prayed, and then I didn't. I tried many different diets, supplements, meditations, you name it. Nothing worked. Our neighbors complained because the concoction I was cooking every day with turtle nails and horse whiskers (not really but something like that) was so strong you could smell it down the hallway in our apartment building. Imagine what that tasted like!

We turned to surrogacy—this at a time when surrogacy was not very common on the East Coast, which was where we lived. There were many problems with our gestational carrier match, and we eventually needed to end the relationship and end the process. We were exhausted and depressed. Our moods were low, and we had very little energy.

My self-esteem was in the toilet. I felt terrible about my body.

If you have been up and down the fertility roller coaster, you know that besides the emotional drain, there can also be a drain on finances and your time. For some, the process is relatively quick, but for others it is long and fraught with difficulties. We were in the second camp.

When I came to the place where I wished for the pain to end, and my desire to become pregnant was outweighed by a desire to parent, I wanted to turn to adoption. Keith wanted to keep trying. Our new marriage was in turmoil. We were both in individual therapy and couple's therapy. Finally, we mended our relationship and decided to adopt. We were sad and exhausted. The world of fertility treatment had been grueling, and now we were starting all over in a different world. And yes, the adoption world had its own challenges, but today, I can say that we wouldn't change our journey because we have the children who were meant to be ours.

Professionally, I have specialized in fertility treatment for more than two decades. I continue to learn every day and share what I have learned with others new to this field. Most of all, I love helping people through the difficult process of family building when getting pregnant "the old-fashioned way" is not an option. It has always been important to me to help create change in a predominantly heterosexual, white male medical field to include the needs of everyone wishing to become a parent.

I know what it is like to struggle, to want a child and not know where to begin. I also know what it feels like to find a new strategy, a shortcut, or a stress-reduction method that works for you. Those moments are gifts, especially when you're worried about making mistakes and feeling desperate to realize your dream.

Mark

My household is one of energies and questions. We have two busy, bouncy, destructive, inquisitive boys—boys without a mother but with two loving parents. We are a family built out of intention and love through the help of many hands and hearts. We are a family built using the assistance of an egg donor and two gestational carriers.

At random times, my two boys will acknowledge that their family is different; at times, they'll complain that they have two dads; at times, their friends say they are lucky. My husband and I regularly talk with them about the very special person who gave some of her very special cells so Daddy and Papa could have a family. While we acknowledge this very special person, they have not asked—yet—who she is.

It was not easy for me to get here. I struggled with coming out, and one of the biggest reasons was that I really wanted to be a father. How could I be a father as a gay man? I came from a very traditional Greek Orthodox background, which meant that I had to move past a typical pathway to parenthood and open my eyes to the fact that being a parent is about loving and wanting a child—and intent. *Intent* means you want this child and you're going to work hard to be the best parent possible. I had to get past the fact that my traditional family that I was raised in did a good job, but my family was going to be raised in a different way, and it would be okay.

Within two months of meeting my future husband, we took a trip together. At that point in time, I was committed to being a single father if necessary, and then he walked into my life. In the midst of a five-hour drive before a long weekend, I let him know that if he did not want to have children, we should not continue to have a relationship. I suggested that we spend the weekend together and then talk about it on the way back. On the return trip, he told me he was on board.

Greg and I started our journey to donor conception with tremendous enthusiasm and excitement. As somebody with many years in the fertility field, I thought we had this. But along the way, we had struggles finding the right donor, and we encountered several hurdles with our surrogacy journey as well. Not only was this roller coaster of hope and disappointment painful for us, but it was also incredibly frustrating. As a fertility doctor, I had been helping people build families for years, but most of these people were not LGBTQIA+ individuals. At that time, there were limited options for people in the LGBTQIA+ community who wanted to become parents. In spite of all the knowledge and experience I had, I couldn't overcome the limitations of our heteronormative culture.

At the same time, I know that I am fortunate. In the 1970s and '80s, being a part of the LGBTQIA+ community was much tougher, and the AIDS epidemic made things beyond complicated. Men had to give up on the idea of having a family to live as their true selves. If it was a struggle for me to become a father, it was a virtual impossibility for earlier generations. Thankfully, this has changed in the United States and many other countries, and it is changing across the world.

I have learned much through my twenty-five years helping others build their families. I also learned a great deal from being the patient, particularly about choosing a donor, perhaps the biggest choice patients face. At its core, choosing a donor might seem like a straightforward task, but there is nothing in the collective intelligence of humanity that ever prepares someone for that. It's a choice imbued with hope and excitement as well as anxiety—and so much more. I advise parents-to-be about their donor choice every day, and it has not gotten easier. In fact, it has gotten more challenging. Thankfully, now there is the opportunity to meet your donor, more genetic information available, and a greater acceptance of family building by LGBTQIA+ individuals.

It took more than two years for my partner and me to get our first family-building journey underway. My hope is that we continue to pave the path for the people who come after us so it will be easier and faster. To this end, I began our fertility clinic, Illume Fertility, and Gay Parents to Be to provide information and great science to help all different families-to-be reach their dreams.

You Are Not Alone

Donor conception, in various forms, has been practiced for longer than we can record. In recent history, there are many documented stories of doctors who inseminated (sometimes with their own sperm) the wives of men who were infertile without their consent, or inseminated women and told them not to tell their children of their origins. When the first egg donor baby was born in Australia in 1983, curiosity about families using this technology increased.[1]

But times are changing—fast. Once shrouded in secrecy, the modern family, built with the assistance of gamete (egg or sperm) donation, is coming out of the shadows and growing exponentially. As more people see friends, family members, and celebrities use donor conception to build their families, the process has become much more mainstream and accepted. Donor sperm programs and egg banks have grown enormously in the past decade, and the news is full of politicians, athletes, and entertainers like Elton John, Anderson Cooper, Andy Cohen, Camille Guaty, and Natalie Imbruglia who have used donor gametes to have their children.

There is not a national registry that tracks the utilization of donors across the country for donors or donor-conceived children, and many people inseminate at home on their own, but several sources report findings that validate the experiences we have every day: The donor market is growing rapidly. The National Institutes of Health provides a "low estimate" of 132,660 sperm donations between 2013 and 2015, and 440,986 between 2015 and 2017 in the United States alone.[2] It is clear that, as a recent report from the UK put it, "Fertility treatment using donor eggs and sperm is on the increase (both IVF and donor insemination)."[3]

Why the increase? At least two factors seem to be playing a role. As more women have entered positions of power, they have felt the loosening of social stigmas and gender stereotypes, and many now feel empowered to become single mothers or delay childbearing. Since a woman's eggs age dramatically in her thirties, women who delay childbearing often find they are not able to use their genetics to conceive and often need to use a donor to build their families.

At the same time, passage of the Marriage Equality Act in 2011 and the legalization of same-sex marriage in all fifty states in 2015 helped create a sense of security for same-sex couples who want to marry and create families. Increasingly, there's a feeling of safety and acceptance of LGBTQIA+ families in our communities. And you can see the results in a recent report from the Family Equality Council that found that more than three million LGBTQIA+ millennials are looking forward to having children[4]—they don't see the barriers that previous generations have seen, and they are aware that they have the option of assisted reproductive technology. There is a national registry that has tracked the utilization of egg donation in male intended parents since 2017, and it has grown year over year. As of 2020, the majority of cycles involving an egg donor and a surrogate were for male intended parents (2017: 48.5 percent; 2018: 54.6 percent; 2019: 59.2 percent; 2020: 61.1 percent).[5]

A Guide to the Practical and the Emotional

Even though donor conception is growing, you are surely well aware that it is not exactly mainstream yet, and if you're like most people starting the process, you may feel like an uninformed outsider. You may have consulted Dr. Google, but unfortunately, there is a lot of conflicting and false information on the internet. You may have gotten information or stories from relatives or friends, but those relatives or friends may not have correct or full information. Layered on top of this lack of knowledge is the fact that your decision to pursue donor conception may be one of last resort—a choice that comes out of suffering coupled with a desire to bring children into your home. Whether you've suffered deeply or your experience has been relatively smooth, everyone who goes through this process will likely need help managing their feelings and their relationships with their partners and with others.

What this means is that in order to successfully navigate the donor-conception process, you need guidance on both the practical and the emotional aspects. This book provides everything you need to know about all the medical processes, the important facts and variables you need to consider when choosing a donor, the important ways you can prepare your body for pregnancy, and other hard facts. You'll also learn tips and strategies for managing emotional challenges that come with this process: managing the pain of infertility, letting go of old goals in favor of new ones, preparing for single parenthood, learning how to choose your donor, dealing with family and friends, handling difficult ethical dilemmas, disclosing to your future child, and more.

Our information and advice are based on the latest research available, but we also rely on our personal experience and our hearts. This is our passion—we've devoted our careers and our lives to it. It's difficult for us to watch people reinvent the wheel or discover important information after it's too late. We wish there had been a manual to help us through our journeys. That's why we wrote this book. We hope it will be your manual.

You'll get the most out of this book if you read it cover to cover, but you can also use it as a reference, flipping to certain sections as needed. You may find that you don't need some sections right now, but you may return to them after your child is born—for example, to hone your child's narrative or revisit ideas about coping with friends and family. Many of the families with whom we meet are curious about "what's next" and how to prepare for it. This is not an outrageous idea. Chapters such as chapter 9, "Disclosure: What Your Child Needs to Know (And Why It's Helpful to Start Practicing Now)," provide a look ahead, but—as the chapter's subtitle implies—we encourage you to read them and start thinking about that future now.

Similarly, you will find that some material is applicable

to everyone, while some sections are specific to heterosexual couples, LGBTQIA+ couples, or single patients separately. These sections are labeled for easy identification. However, while these sections provide information and guidance that's geared toward specific audiences, you may want to at least skim them all. All people are different, and you may find information that applies to your situation in different sections. Use what you need.

Scattered throughout all these chapters, you will find patient stories, real-life examples of people who have been through donor conception. These stories can provide ideas for how to cope with different challenges, examples of how people have made decisions like those you will have to make, and new ways of seeing your donor-conception journey. Most of all, these stories present a wide range of people—some who will be similar to you in a lot of ways, some who will be totally different—all of whom have "been there." Once again: You are not alone. Although the identities of these patients have been obscured and sometimes are composites of multiple patients, all of them are true to life and based on real patients we have seen. Helping these parents-to-be has been a life's passion for us, and we hope to help you.

Love and Intention Make a Family

The profile of the American family is changing. We have been fortunate to witness and be part of the creation of many single-parent, LGBTQIA+, and multi-parent families, and each one has reaffirmed that love and intention make a family. We hope that you, in spite of any obstacles you may have faced, push ahead with love and intention to create the family you desire. One person may feel their family is full with one child, and another may feel that unless they have three children, their family is not complete. An ideal situation for some may be to use a friend or sibling as a donor, and for others, that would be a total disaster. Everyone deserves to feel fulfilled and whole with the family they desire. The most important thing you can do now is to think about the family you want to have.

Our job is to help you create that family and help you avoid regret. It's what we do. It's all we do. And we never get tired of seeing people like you get through this complicated, often overwhelming process and become a parent.

Part I

||||||||||||||||||||||||||||||||||||||||||||||||||||||||||||||||||||||||||||||||||||||||||||||||||||||||||

Transitioning to Donor Conception

1

Accepting Donor Conception

Donor conception can be a wonderful way to build a family, but it's rarely anyone's first choice. Most couples and individuals would choose to have a baby using only their own genetics if they could. That's natural. Using the genetics of a stranger does feel uncomfortable to many of the people we see. Some parents-to-be who have used donor conception say it can feel like having a ghost in the room. That doesn't mean it's negative—just different. We can relate to this. We've both felt a deep desire to know more about our children's genetic relatives as we watch our children grow up. It creates a feeling of longing, and it makes us work harder to be the best parents we can be.

There's a saying in the adoption world that counselors

and agencies use when talking with people who are considering adoption: You need to make the unfamiliar familiar. If it was your dream to have a baby genetically related to you, shifting to adoption is going to take some getting used to. The same is true of donor conception.

If you're reading this, you've likely chosen to use a donor, or you're seriously considering it. Your decision may be difficult or relatively easy, but either way, choosing to live with the genetics of someone other than you in your child takes a big leap of faith. You are choosing to be a parent. Many people try to make that leap easier by choosing a donor they find attractive, they admire, or who reminds them of themselves, hoping that this will help counteract their feelings of disconnect from that ghost in their family. People often tell us they feel a connection to a donor, or they feel he or she is "the one." Many are not even aware they're doing this; they just want someone with whom they can connect and feel comfortable. We'll talk more about donor choice in part 2, but suffice it to say that your journey through donor conception will be smoother—and much more beneficial for all involved—if you learn as much as you can about the process and understand the implications of this decision for you and your future children. It is important to feel good about your donor choice, but it's also important to be practical. Our desire is for you to build your family and have the easiest journey with the fewest speed bumps and hurdles possible. With no regrets.

The first thing to know is that you *will* be a family, in all the most important ways. You will have the same hopes, dreams, and joys as other parents. You will love and nurture your child, and that child will exhaust and frustrate you like all children do. You will celebrate milestones and face challenges together. Your family will fill you up. It is true you will need to work hard, dig deep, and be hopeful to make this dream come to life, but your efforts will be well worth it.

Obviously, having a child through donor conception is not the same as having a child who is fully genetically linked to two parents, so your family will be different, too. Not *bad* different, just different. Your family will bear the additional responsibility of having your child in a different way. Your child will need a solid sense of self, to know they were wanted and how they came to life, literally—that is, you will need to share frequently that there is a very special person who helped bring them to your family. You will need to be prepared to answer questions they may have about a range of things, including IVF, your donor, and more. You'll have to explain to them that they were loved and wanted even before they came into existence. In my family, I (Mark) have had to field questions that were generated by my son's preschool class when someone there said that he must have a mother and that he must be adopted. If you decide that donor conception is right for you, this difference is something you will get used to as you realize the love of a child is greater than the love one may have for their own genetics. We have often said to our patients that if someone dropped a baby off at your door, no matter how much the child did or did not look like you, you would take care of that child and fall hopelessly in love. Human beings have an incredible capacity to love and nurture.

And we promise you this: While the effort you put into building your family and nurturing your family may seem daunting, it gets easier over time. It's been said that most of a rocket's fuel is burned during takeoff. If you are beginning this journey, you may feel like you're burning a *lot* of fuel, but donor conception won't feel so daunting, anxiety producing, or scary forever. One day, it will be a part of you and your family. That rocket will be cruising.

People come to donor conception through one of three paths: heterosexual couples diagnosed with one of the many causes of infertility, LGBTQIA+ couples desiring to have a child, or individuals who choose to be single parents. We have helped create thousands of happy families from each of these groups. While your own story is unique, it's our hope that reading about people in similar situations will help you feel less alone as you come to terms with your decision to use a donor.

Infertility

ANA

Ana had gotten pregnant three times over the past couple of years, but each time, she miscarried within the first couple of months. After a fertility workup and a few unsuccessful IVF cycles, it was determined that she was unlikely to have success using her own eggs. Her doctor suggested she and her husband, John, consider using egg donation to have a child. When she came to the Center for Family Building, she and John were quarreling every day, and Ana believed her marriage might fall apart. To make things worse, her younger sister was seven months pregnant, and her baby shower was coming up. "I want to feel happy for her, but I can't and I feel terrible," Ana told me (Lisa). She pulled her sweater cuffs down over her fists as she spoke. "I'm the older sister; I was supposed to have children first. I'm so upset, and John just doesn't understand why I feel so sad all the time. Before I was diagnosed with infertility, I would have loved the idea of being an aunt to her baby, but now I just don't think I can take it. I can't deal with her baby bump, all the comments from my family about how excited they all are, and I know they will ask me to host the shower. How am I going to handle all of this?"

In counseling, Ana worked hard to learn new stress-reduction techniques to help her withstand the stressors of treatment and in her life. She worked on her relationship with her husband and found a way to manage her interactions with her sister and her family so she could preserve her relationships while also protecting her heart. She knew she wouldn't have a child overnight and was willing to employ strategies to get her through this difficult time in her life.

As you might imagine—and as you might have experienced—Ana's sadness and pain are not unusual. Infertility can cause anxiety, a drop in self-esteem, and depression. In fact, research has shown that infertility patients can experience depressive feelings similar to those felt by cancer patients.[1]

It's no wonder. From the time we are young, we understand that babies are made by people, and for many, eventually becoming a parent feels like a given. We may look up to our own parents and want to emulate them. We may play with dolls or see others play with dolls. We may even fantasize about the family we want to have. We are surrounded by families, and most people assume that getting pregnant is the easiest thing in the world. The menstrual cycle is the monthly evidence that a woman's body is built to have babies, and as heterosexual people get older and become sexually active, they are often keenly aware of birth control and how *not* to get pregnant. Naturally, when infertility or a medical condition makes childbirth—this basic principle of life—unlikely for someone, the hurt that causes can be devastating. This idea that something is "wrong" can feel enormously painful. And the world can feel like it's caving in.

The pain and grief created by infertility can be accompanied by frustration, anger, and resentment. Sometimes one or both people in a relationship may direct these feelings at their partner—for delaying family-building plans, for not being available for treatment appointments, or for not following medical advice by not eating or having sex the way the doctor has prescribed. Conflict in the relationship can deepen your hurt and depression. Often in heterosexual relationships, we see men and women reacting differently to infertility, particularly when there is a female factor issue. We see men take a more optimistic position, believing everything will turn out fine as long as they follow their doctor's directions. Women, on the other hand, often feel anxious and sad. They want to plan ahead for each step in the process, they worry that they might be doing something wrong, and they feel eager to fix the problem. Unfortunately, there are a lot of unknowns and a lot of waiting in fertility treatment. This can intensify a woman's anxiety because there is little to do once her doctor sets course on her treatment plan. If you're feeling these feelings, please know that you are not alone. It can feel maddening to not be in the driver's seat and to feel like no one understands your pain—even your partner. If your husband sees things differently from the way you do, it's not necessarily a comment on his commitment to become parents or his love for you. It's just that when it comes to infertility, two people in a couple can react very differently. And that's okay as long as you're able to accept it and find ways to manage it so the infertility does not eat away at your relationship.

It is also important for heterosexual couples to understand that sometimes the tables are turned. Men can have genetic disorders, anatomic disorders, or trauma that prevents them from ever being a genetic father. These men suffer a tremendous amount of grief and loss. If we consider that men never get a chance to be pregnant and a lot of "being a man" in our society is tied up in the idea of passing on a legacy in the form of a child, this can be especially traumatic. It can absolutely lead to issues of self-loathing and relationship avoidance. But these men often do choose to put their desire to be a father over the need to use their genetics. It takes work, but it is regularly done.

To make matters worse, oftentimes people turn their angry feelings against themselves. When people suffer from infertility, it can affect their self-esteem. You may blame yourself for any number of things, criticize your decisions or your body for not performing the way it should, or conclude that you are simply unlucky or destined to live without children. Some of our patients with infertility tell us they think their partners should leave them. This drop in self-esteem is a hallmark of infertility. And these attacks at the self are also likely to create more depression and anxiety.[2] [3]

The infertility journey is often called a roller coaster, and for good reason. The cycles of hope and disappointment can cause stress and depression, and this can be overwhelming. Many people find it hard to focus at work, be available for friends, or even have sex with their partner. Outsiders often cannot understand or even imagine these feelings, and so they may be unsupportive. Therefore, infertility patients can feel misunderstood and disconnected from the people upon whom they typically depend. Unfortunately, isolation can cause depression to worsen.

Losses are also common in the process of infertility treatment. These can include pregnancy losses or a failed cycle. They can also include the shock of the beginning of a new menstrual cycle, the sadness of your best friend getting pregnant first, or watching friends or people on social media have the families you thought you would have by now. When the idea of donor conception is broached, the pain and grief are once again exacerbated. Many people feel dread as they mentally add up more losses, even as they may not even realize the number of losses that are accumulating inside them. The loss of a genetic connection. The loss of a dream. The loss of a tie to one's heritage or family name. The loss of creating a child with the person you love and experiencing the joy of looking for each other's traits in that child. Then there are losses about things like the due date and the baby names. These thoughts and fantasies are all part of the big dream of having a child, and they can all come crashing down when those dreams are lost.

People often feel shock as well. They may say, "What about my best friend who got pregnant at forty-two? Or what about Janet Jackson?" Celebrities, and sometimes good friends, may not be open about using donor conception to build their families. Unfortunately, this lack of openness has caused more people to delay parenthood because of the perception that it's not so hard to successfully give birth at an older age. It has also contributed to more secrecy around donor conception—and with secrecy comes shame, which can compound the hurt of infertility and make moving to donor conception even harder. Perhaps someday we will see more famous donor-conceived children telling their stories in the media and erasing the needless shame.

Then there is worry. *Will I care for my child in the same way I would if we were genetically connected? Will my child care for me as deeply as she might if we were genetically connected? And what will others think? Will they judge us? Will they see this child as my child? Will knowing my child is donor-conceived change their relationship with them? Will my child be looked at differently by their friends or teachers?* You may also be worried about having genetic relatives of your child in the world. The donor and donor-related siblings are out there and will always be a genetic link to your future child. You may worry about whether your child will have a relationship with these people and what those relationships will look like. Will it be overwhelming or difficult? Will it affect their sense of self?

These are some of the worries experienced by Ana, the woman profiled at the beginning of this section. She also worried that the child may love John more than her because they would be genetically connected. She worried that she might not love the child as much if she didn't share genetics with them. She worried that she was depriving her parents from having a grandchild that would carry on their family line. They were immigrants and proud of their culture, and now that culture could be lost forever. Ana lost sleep over these worries. She wanted to talk to her friends about it but was worried they would judge her. After all the fertility treatments, she had a tough transition toward the thought of using a donor to conceive. The idea seemed almost impossible at first. It wasn't until she learned more about donor conception by working with her clinic that she began to feel more comfortable with the idea.

One more thing to consider is that this is a time when you may be feeling stress from two different sources. You hold loss and grief about not having a child and loss and grief about not being able to have a genetic tie to your future child. In the same place. These two sets of emotions are so intertwined that they may feel like one, but they are not. When you have your baby, the pain of being childless will be gone. You will be a parent. You will have joy and so many fantastic experiences as a family.

However, some of those feelings about not having a genetically linked child may remain. Will they fade over time? Yes. They will become part of you, and just like other losses in your life, the sting will fade and you will become more comfortable with the new life you have created. If you are beginning your journey, it may be hard to imagine that you will become more comfortable with it. But if donor conception is right for you, like it was for Ana, you can become more comfortable and embrace it over time. And the more you learn, the more grounded you can feel in managing the process, and that can give you a great deal of solace. In fact, you may even begin to grow more warmth and gratitude toward your donor, because this is the person who helped you become a parent.

None of this means it will never bother you again. It may. One day, you may be in the supermarket with your daughter when a stranger says, "Oh, your daughter looks exactly like you," and your heart will sink. You may think, *Wow, I forgot,* or, *Ooh, that still hurts a bit.* But you will look at your child, whom you adore, and be so grateful she is yours, even if you don't share genetics. Remember, even in traditional families there are children who do not look like one parent or another, and many siblings do not look anything like each other. This is an expression of fifty-two thousand individual genes being rolled on the great craps table known as nature. There are more than seven billion of us on the planet, and none of us are the same. It's important to keep genetics in perspective.

So how do you get there? Time. And everyone needs a different amount of it. As we said above, education helps a lot. The fact that you picked up this book means you are on your way to a decision that is right for you. Processing your feelings with a reproductive counselor can also be extremely helpful. It can help you feel supported and help you absorb the reality of using donor conception to have a child. When people engage in therapy with a counselor who specializes in this area, they typically feel more resolved and prepared when their child is born.

I (Lisa) once worked with a woman in our clinic who said, "If I make a cake using a cake mix or if I make a cake from scratch, it will taste the same." This woman felt that becoming a parent was more important than having a genetic connection to a child. Donor conception was not her first choice, and she was shocked and saddened when she learned she could not use her genetics to build her family, but using her genetics did not hold as much weight for her as it does for others.

For others, the choice is much harder.

VANESSA

Vanessa struggled to accept using donor eggs. Throughout treatment, she worried. Throughout her pregnancy, she worried. One of her biggest concerns was that she wouldn't feel a strong connection to her donor-conceived children (she was pregnant with twins). We worked on these concerns and the meaning they had for her. When she had her children, a boy and a girl, she gave them the names she had planned for them, but she had a nagging, uncomfortable feeling about her daughter's name. She later changed her daughter's name and finally felt a more solid connection to her child.

Sometimes women do feel disconnected from their unborn children while pregnant. We have worked with several of these women over the years.

And perhaps Vanessa would have felt the same way about any girl she had at first. There is no way to know. What we do know is that Vanessa has always been thoughtful and considerate of her children, speaks openly with them about their donor, and feels very grateful to this woman who helped her become a parent. She has a lovely story about her donor and is open to her children meeting her when they desire. Though it took her time to get there, Vanessa is comfortable with donor conception.

These are extreme examples. Most people find their transition happens somewhere between those two points. What is important to know is that it happens. In more than two decades of seeing donor-conception recipients, we have rarely seen a parent who wanted to have a child, chose donor conception, and wasn't able to eventually embrace it.

Acceptance usually happens in stages. When heterosexual couples are trying to conceive at home, they often think, *I could never use fertility treatment,* until they do. Or *I could never use intrauterine insemination,* until they do. Or, what feels like taking out the big guns for many, *I could never use in vitro fertilization.* But they do.

It's true that donor conception is a big leap, and most people don't take that leap and land with both feet on the ground, fully accepting it. If you have someone knowledgeable to shepherd you along, you are less likely to get stuck on one of these "nevers" or other difficulties. It is our hope that this book can help you on your journey.

A short note about fate. Many people believe that if God or fate or whatever you believe in wanted them to have a child, they would have one. If this is your perspective, we completely honor it. Another way to look at it, however, is that God (or nature) gave us the ability to make medical interventions. For example, many of us have been vaccinated against mumps, rubella, influenza, and COVID. Some may say those things are life-threatening, which makes them necessary, unlike having a donor-conceived baby. But what about getting braces on your teeth when they are crooked or taking supplements to improve your health? What about getting a root canal to improve your oral health, or taking novocaine so you won't feel the pain of that root canal? These can be considered "quality of life" decisions, and most of us make them without batting an eyelash. Our society utilizes modern medicine on a daily basis to bring life into the world, prevent disease, preserve life, and correct physical abnormalities. Science and medicine are available to help you build your family if you so choose.

One more thing that may be helpful is a closure cycle. Many of our patients find they can more easily move on to donor conception if they try one last time to get pregnant through fertility treatment. Something about trying just one more time can feel reassuring. For some, this final attempt gives them confirmation that donor conception is "meant to be." For others, it is simply confirmation that what they have been doing is not working, and that helps them start to close the chapter of genetic parenthood and perhaps, even if it's just a crack, open up the possibility of parenthood through donor conception. If this is important to you, you should honor that feeling and discuss it with your doctor.

It can feel empowering, especially when so much of trying to conceive feels out of control, to have solid information to help you feel better and even possibly avoid regret. It is a terrible feeling to keep wondering, *What would have happened if I had tried once more?* We have talked about the importance of educating yourself so you will know you are doing all you can to make the best choices for you, your partner, and your future child, and a closure cycle can be part of that education. If you have the coverage for this option or can afford it, it can be a helpful step in moving forward to donor conception.

LGBTQIA+ Couples

JAMAL AND CURT

Jamal and Curt wanted two children, one from each of their genetics. But when they learned about the high cost of having two pregnancies with a gestational carrier, they decided that perhaps they would have one child, but to connect their child to both of their genetics, they would use eggs donated by

Curt's sister and fertilize them with Jamal's sperm. They were very excited they had a plan again, but then they ran into another problem. After Curt's sister was assessed, they learned that she was not a good candidate for egg donation.

This saddened them, but they understood that using Curt's sister as an egg donor would probably not yield any good embryos, and they would need to start over. After talking about it with us and on their own, they changed their plan once again: They decided to use a nonidentified (or anonymous) donor with each of their sperm. They were concerned about the expense of donor eggs, but they were determined to make it work.

The next question they faced was whose genetics they would use first. They could freeze embryos with both of their sperm and first use an embryo from one partner, and later, if they could afford it, come back and use an embryo created with the other partner's sperm. But if they only ended up having one child, one of them would not have a genetically linked child. After talking about it in counseling and with their respective families, they learned that Jamal's aunt on his dad's side had a significant mental illness. While the genetic risk was not big, they had to choose. So they decided to use Curt's embryos to have a child first, and if they later decided to have a second child, they would consider using Jamal's embryos.

The couple soon had a beautiful baby boy, but not before resolving several obstacles along the way. It took a lot of talking, a lot of patience, and a strong commitment to each other and to the idea of having a family.

Over the course of our careers, the challenges and struggles that LGBTQIA+ couples face in family building have been shrinking and changing dramatically. For many years, folks in the queer community wondered if they could be parents at all. When I (Lisa) began lecturing at LGBTQIA+ centers about reproductive options in the late 1990s, I would be fortunate to have an audience of four. Ten years later, an audience of one hundred was not surprising. Today, we see LGBTQIA+ individuals and couples every day in our practices.

When I (Mark) created Gay Parents to Be, it was a passion project. Now, it is a busy hub for education, connection, and support through family building. Whereas I struggled to get past my own coming-out process and internalized homophobia to build a family, at this point, more than 70 percent of my practice is LGBTQIA+. I am regularly buoyed and inspired by the young people I see who are moving forward with their lives, building their families, and being extremely thoughtful about choosing their donor and how they will speak to their child. Many of these LGBTQIA+ parents-to-be have been together since their twenties and are deciding to have children in their thirties, just like any fertile heterosexual couple. Truly a paradigm shift in the past thirty years. This paradigm shift has happened in my lifetime and inspires me to keep helping our community. Our families provide visibility and validation for our entire community.

Marriage equality, gay celebrities having babies, and the first gay family on the cover of *Parents* magazine in 2019 have all helped move the needle on normalizing queer parenthood. However, there are still obstacles and feelings of stress, disappointment, and hurt. Our patients describe a range of struggles, from the unfairness of the medical or insurance system to the enormous cost of treatment, from confusion about the medical process to the time and energy involved in making it all happen. And for many, there is the basic pain of not being able to "just try at home."

Perhaps because our culture still tends to default to the heteronormative, some queer couples also find it difficult to fully feel entitled to parenthood. While this is changing, sometimes queer parents-to-be have concerns, like, *How will my child cope without a mother (or father)? Will the world accept us as parents? If we have an opposite-sex child, will we know what to do?* Add to that the stress of learning a medical process that can feel brain twisting, countless doctors' appointments and legal forms, hurrying up just to wait for a donor or an agency, a feeling of a loss of control in treatment, experiencing the effects of hormones, or—when using a gestational carrier—a feeling of not having enough control and having to rely on the decisions of another for the health of your child. It can feel like a lot to handle.

For trans parents-to-be, it is typically even more complicated. Ceasing hormones can cause an emotional setback and lead to physical changes, and the reminders of your assigned sex at birth, which can feel very upsetting and trigger past traumatic experiences. Providing a sperm sample or having a genital exam can cause feelings of sadness or embarrassment. This is a subject for a much longer discussion, and this is only the very tip of the iceberg, but suffice it to say, family building can be very challenging for trans individuals or couples.

And if your clinic is not queer-friendly, you may face daily upsets. Your doctor may use the wrong name or pronoun, and your paperwork may exclude you or misrepresent you. Bathrooms, procedures, and office materials may cater to heterosexual folks only, and your doctor may be in the dark about how to best treat you, ask you the right questions, and warmly guide you on your path to parenthood. There are many groups, such as the Human Rights Campaign, the Family Equality Council, and Lambda Legal, that can guide you and provide you with information to help you make legal and medical decisions on your family-building journey.

Queer couples typically don't feel the same pain as those with infertility; they have a different kind of pain. We are different, and our family-building challenges are significant. All these challenges can make it difficult for some to accept donor conception. On top of that, you share the same need with infertility patients to accept that someone else, someone outside your relationship, will be contributing to your family—a person who may feel like a stranger to you. Although you are not literally bringing that person into your home, their genetics will be part of your child, and that can feel uncomfortable to many.

When there is no choice but to choose a donor to have a child, many people naturally look for someone who feels comfortable or familiar to them. While familiar traits can play a role in donor choice, you may find that simply becoming educated about how to make the best choice for you can play a big role in helping you accept donor conception. You'll read more about donor choice later in this book. Even though you can't simply get pregnant at home (hopefully one day we will find a way to make that work), you can thoughtfully choose the best donor for your family, and that can feel very grounding and calming.

For LGBTQIA+ patients, holding your child in your arms represents a dream that you may never have thought could come true. It is a cathartic moment in which you will experience a new kind of love: that of a child.

Single Parents-to-Be

HANNAH

A lovely, smart, and personable thirty-two-year-old woman, Hannah met with us determined to pursue single parenthood. She had been in a relationship for many years with a man who had children from a previous relationship and did not want more. Hannah thought she would feel okay not having children of her own, but as she moved past thirty, her desire to have a child grew. "Soon I realized that I would regret it for the rest of my life if I didn't have one," she told me (Lisa) later, smiling ruefully.

Hannah left her boyfriend and leaped into treatment. She did it all. Acupuncture and nutrition to improve her ability to conceive. Counseling for stress management. Single mothers' groups. You name it, there was no stone unturned—she was all in. During counseling, she discussed how she would manage as a single mother, how she could care for a child alone with little family support, whether she was "right" to have a child without a partner, and all the issues involved in parenting a donor-conceived child. She chose her sperm donor, and she felt highly prepared.

Then the bottom dropped out. Intrauterine insemination didn't work. In vitro fertilization didn't work. Finally, her doctor recommended ovum donation. Initially, Hannah said, "I have no problem using an egg donor," and began her search. She learned about the open donor program we have at Illume and decided to choose an open donor. Things seemed to be moving ahead nicely, but then one day, she canceled her doctor's appointment. And then she canceled her next doctor's appointment. And then Hannah halted her treatment. After her long journey, she decided not to continue the process for the time being. She realized that she was more attached to her genetics than she had thought.

PETER

Peter is a gay man who came out in college but never dated much. He was a focused student, and he went on to become a successful physician. Soon after launching his career, he had his first meaningful relationship. When the relationship ended after five years, Peter found himself wanting a child more than another relationship. He told us that he wanted to marry one day, but he felt unsure about when that would happen. "I want to have a child while I'm still young," he said. His parents had had Peter later in life, and he wanted them to enjoy a grandchild. Also, he wanted to share his child with his large extended family. So Peter took on the task of family building without a partner. We helped provide a supportive environment and helped him through his journey, and his family was supportive. At first, Peter's parents pushed him to choose a donor who looked like she "belonged" in the family, but Peter, after carefully considering his options, chose the most practical choice—one whose genetics would provide a better chance for a healthy baby. His parents, being loving parents, eventually decided that Peter's choice looked just like many of their family members after all. His cousin agreed to be the gestational carrier. Three years later, Peter is still single but very happy—and busy with his beautiful toddler.

Though people who intentionally choose to be a single parent represent the smallest group of patients, we both see single people planning to have children every week. At Illume Fertility, we have a single mothers' program. I (Mark) have been talking to single men about family building since long before single male celebrities such as TV journalist Anderson Cooper, soccer star Cristiano Ronaldo, and TV host and producer Andy Cohen elevated it in the public dialogue. Some of these patients once hoped that they would build their family with a partner, while others feel that a family of two is just perfect. Sometimes we see individuals planning to parent with the assistance of their own parents, while others want to parent solo.

Decades ago, it was unheard of to choose to be a single mother. After all, it was unlikely a woman could support a child alone, and society used to label women who reached a certain age as "old maids." And stereotypes about men and women may have prevented many men from having children alone. We've come a long way since then. Still, while there is much less shame and fewer roadblocks to single parenthood than there used to be, the problems that accompany having a child alone have not completely evaporated. In many places in the world, including some communities in the United States, we see prejudice prevent people from having the children they desire. In many cases, cultural or religious differences cause family members, teachers, or even the parents at soccer practice to whisper and gossip. You may have prepared well financially and practically, but that doesn't mean it will not be difficult to be pregnant, choose a donor, or go through treatment alone.

Although it is a cliché, it is also true: It does take a village to raise a child. If you are a single parent-to-be, we encourage you to use all the resources at your disposal. Support organizations such as Single Mothers by Choice can be tremendously helpful, but so can your religious institution, your book club, or your neighbors. All of these can help you in both practical and emotional ways, from picking up dinner to accompanying you to doctors' appointments to watching the baby while you take a nap. The modern family is very different from the families most of us knew when we were young. It can consist of one parent and several uncles and aunts or friends and relatives. Simply because you are parenting alone, that doesn't mean you need to parent alone. You can construct your unique family and support system. We can construct our chosen family. Part of growing up is making the decision of who will be your supports and who, regardless of their relationship to you, you know you cannot rely on. You may be very resilient and be able to power through everything you need to do to create your family, but don't underestimate the power of help or a hug or a pat on the shoulder. It does wonders to fill up your emotional fuel tank.

What is most important is that you carefully explore your desires and think thoroughly through the ramifications of your decisions. Also, remember you are human. Remember Hannah? She has put family building on the shelf. She decided to change jobs and now wants to date. Hannah still wants to be a mom, but since she now will use donor sperm and donor eggs, there is no rush. Not using her genetics was a big change for her, and she wants time to settle in with it—and maybe even not do it alone after all. Peter, on the other hand, had an easier time with the process and is thrilled with his life with his daughter. Although some of these stories may resonate with you, everyone is different. At different parts of your journey, *you* may feel different. That is okay. You need to find the path that works for you, and fortunately, we are now living in a world where there are many options.

Whether you are choosing a donor because of infertility, because you're in a same-sex relationship, or because you are choosing single parenthood, the child you will create will be your child 100 percent. Your donor is not asking to parent the child (unless you are co-parenting). They want to help you have a child of your own. In this moment in time, you and the donor are focused on contributing to a new life, but then you will each refocus on your own lives. This does not mean you cannot have an open relationship if you want one or reach out to a donor who is willing to connect in the future, because those things are possible, especially with an egg donation. It does mean that when you have a child, you will be going to parent-teacher meetings and soccer games, kissing boo-boos, and getting up in the middle of the night when your child is sick or has a nightmare. And you will be forever intricately connected to a new human being in a way that you are not connected to anyone else in the world.

2

How Does This Work?

We're guessing that you have a pretty good idea of how "this" works—where *this* refers to how babies are made. Sperm meets egg. Sperm fertilizes egg. Egg becomes embryo. Embryo becomes fetus becomes baby. A beautiful story.

When it comes to donor conception, the story is more complicated but no less beautiful. In fact, even after decades in the field, we still find it deeply moving and utterly fantastical. It is sometimes difficult to believe that there are all these wonderful ways that life can be brought into this world. We never tire of witnessing these miracles and feel privileged to cooperate with nature to help people build the families of their dreams.

Whether you are using donated sperm, donated eggs, or donated embryos, the donor-conception process begins with choosing your donor, a decision that is exciting but also can feel overwhelming and emotional. Part 2 will walk you through everything you need to know to make the best decision for you, so you can feel confident and comfortable moving forward to the donation. Once you've chosen your donor, you are ready to proceed with the donation. How that looks to you will depend on which gamete you are having donated. We'll start with sperm.

Using Donor Sperm

Patients using donor sperm might be a couple in which the male partner has no sperm or a very low sperm count, a single female, or a same-sex female couple. Prior to insemination, the female recipient, or person with the uterus, will work with a medical professional to prepare for conception. You will undergo uterine testing and may use your natural cycle or take medication to prepare the uterine lining (preparation and testing are discussed in detail in chapter 3). If you are prescribed medication to grow and multiply the number of eggs you have available for the cycle, you will take those medications for five days to two weeks before the eggs are ready to be fertilized. During that time, you will visit the clinic for blood work and ultrasounds so your doctor can make sure all is going well and your eggs are growing in number and size. When your doctor determines that an egg is about to be released, you'll be asked to go to the office and have an insemination.

Your clinic will be prepared to warm the vial of sperm of your chosen donor, each of which is expected to have five to ten million mobile sperm within it. These vials have been cryopreserved after donation, but when you arrive at the clinic, an andrologist—a scientist who works with sperm—will take one vial out, slowly warm it, assess it for viability and count, and place it in a solution compatible with the female reproductive tract, all to get it ready for you.

An insemination is similar to a Pap smear in that the doctor places a speculum within the vagina. The doctor then gently cleans the cervix, inserts a small tube through the cervix, and releases the sperm at the top of the uterine cavity using a syringe. There is no needle involved. In a typical insemination, you will receive a specimen of about 0.5 milliliters, or one-tenth of a teaspoon. After insertion, millions of sperm will pass to the end of the fallopian tube to "greet" the about-to-be-released egg. The egg is released from the ovary and picked up by the end of the fallopian tube, where hundreds of thousands of sperm surround it. The procedure takes five to ten minutes, and you may feel some mild discomfort and cramping while it is happening.

While common wisdom says it takes one sperm to make a baby, the reality is that it takes tens of thousands of sperm to fertilize one egg. This is because the egg is surrounded by a jelly mass, and the sperm is equipped with enzymes to break down this jelly mass. Slowly, they do that as a group until they reach the shell of the egg. The one sperm that gets through the shell of the egg and meets the membrane of the egg first ends up causing a release of calcium in the membrane of the egg, which acts as a force field and blocks any other sperm from piercing the membrane of the egg. That is nature's way of making sure only a single sperm fertilizes an egg.

After the insemination, there isn't much to do except wait ten to sixteen days for a pregnancy test. We recommend healthy lifestyle choices and self-nurturing during this time. You are allowed to exercise and follow your normal routine. I (Mark) always say to my patients, "Sperm float, fallopian tubes float; just go about your normal life." What's happening in your body is sperm is meeting eggs, and we hope that fertilization as described above is happening and an embryo is created. If it is, that embryo will travel down your fallopian tube over a period of four to seven days to reach your uterine cavity. By the time it reaches your uterine cavity, that embryo is now a blastocyst, which is the first major differentiation stage of a human embryo. Instead of being one ball of cells, there are now two types of cells within the embryo. A group of cells called the *inner cell mass* is the group that will become the fetus. Surrounding the inner cell mass is a group called the *trophectoderm cells,* which will eventually become the placenta. Another way to think of a blastocyst is to picture a daisy, where the center (yellow) part is the part that makes the embryo, and the petals of the flower are the part that allows for implantation in the uterus. It really is quite remarkable that after five to seven days of embryonic development, cell lines have differentiated to define which cells will become the embryo and which will become the placenta, which is a natural phenomenon biologically programmed by our human genetic code, or if you prefer, a higher power.

While you wait, you have a whole team of professionals waiting with you and rooting for your success. It can be a time of hope and anxiety for you. In reproductive medicine, it is common knowledge that the "two-week wait," or some variation of that, can feel like torture to patients. You may feel out of control and stressed, watching each hour drag on, waiting for that pregnancy test. This is a great time to practice stress management (we provide some techniques in chapter 11), especially the techniques that provide you with a sense of control.

As a side note, different physicians will give you many different answers about how much exercise you can do during this time. We have all heard of people who were going to the gym or training for a marathon when they discovered they were several weeks pregnant, so it's likely that some exercise will be fine for you as well. However, I (Lisa) often tell patients that if, heaven forbid, you discover you are not pregnant or you lose the pregnancy, you don't want to wonder if it was because of that run on the treadmill or the push-ups or crunches you did after your transfer. If you're someone who enjoys going to the gym or uses vigorous exercise for stress relief, it can be especially challenging to hold off, but you may want to think about whether it's worth it to you—not because it will likely cause a problem but because the possible self-recrimination is terrible.

Some patients who use donated sperm will have an in

vitro fertilization procedure (or IVF, fertilization that is conducted outside the body) instead of an insemination. This option is typically the best one for women who are older, because it gives us the opportunity to select the embryos we use. Think of it this way: The eggs in a woman's body can be compared to the balls inside a bingo cage. When you're eighteen years old, your bingo cage is filled with white balls—good, healthy eggs. But as you get older, a few red balls get mixed into the cage. Those represent the less viable eggs—the ones that likely won't lead to a successful conception. The older a woman gets, the more red balls she has in that cage. When you spin the cage and pull the lever, you don't know if you'll get a red or a white ball. But with IVF, you skip the lever altogether. IVF gives you the opportunity to go into the cage, grab a handful of balls, fertilize all of them with sperm, and see which embryos are more likely to be viable.

If you undergo IVF instead of an insemination, your eggs will be harvested in a small surgical procedure. You will likely be given anesthesia for the procedure and will be asked to take that day off from work. Although you will be at the clinic for some time to prep and recover, the actual procedure takes only twenty to thirty minutes, and no incision is necessary. Most patients have a bit of cramping or spotting afterward (our bodies just don't love being poked, but they recover pretty quickly). But if you take the day off, relax, maybe enjoy some bad TV, and sleep off the medication, you should feel fine to go back to work the next day.

After your eggs have been retrieved, they will be fertilized in the lab with the donor sperm you have chosen. Again, you will have an anxious period of waiting to see if embryos develop. At Illume Fertility, you will receive a phone call the next day to confirm fertilization, another call two days later to define embryonic growth, and a call four days later to see how many blastocysts have formed. Different practices manage this information stream differently, but you will be updated about your embryonic development. If you are having a fresh embryo transfer, you'll return to the clinic approximately five days after your egg retrieval to have an embryo carefully transferred to your uterus. Egg retrieval, fertilization, and transfer are all covered in the next section.

Using Donor Eggs

Some of the most common patients seeking donor conception are women who want to be parents but whose own quality or quantity of eggs has declined, often with aging, and they are no longer able to become pregnant with their own eggs. For these women, using donor eggs will give them their best chance of having a healthy baby. Single males and same-sex male couples make up the remainder of patients who use donated eggs. As with patients using donated sperm, one of the first things all these patients need to do is choose a donor. In this case, you may choose a donor who will undergo a stimulation cycle so that her eggs can be retrieved and fertilized with sperm, or you can use eggs that were previously retrieved from a donor and are now frozen.

Egg Banks and Fresh Donors

In the past, the only donor eggs available were fresh donor eggs, which have been used in IVF since 1983. Over the years, advances in cryopreservation methods allowed for the successful freezing of unfertilized eggs, and in recent years, the use of previously frozen eggs has grown in popularity. There are advantages and disadvantages to both fresh and frozen eggs.

If you choose to use frozen eggs from an egg bank, you will typically receive six to eight eggs in a batch, which is fewer than you will typically get from a donation of fresh eggs. Frozen eggs need to survive thawing, which can reduce their number. When the eggs are fertilized, it reduces their number further. Depending on how many eggs are successfully fertilized, patients using frozen eggs often end up with only enough embryos for one attempt at embryo transfer and a child. Some egg banks have some version of a guarantee program, but often one lot or batch of eggs is what you will receive for a fixed price—period. Donors of frozen eggs are considered anonymous, in that no identifying information is shared between the recipient and the donor (though as we will discuss later, anonymity is impossible in this era of at-home genetic testing). There are some egg banks that are now giving an option of future contact from the child when they become an adult.

Cryopreservation

Cryopreservation, or freezing, has been used in medicine for more than fifty years, and it is a safe process. The technique of cryopreservation in modern fertility laboratories is called *vitrification,* which involves adding sugar molecules to the media that are absorbed by the embryos to stabilize the high water content within them. This makes them more tolerant of extreme temperatures and allows them to avoid ice formation, which would rupture and break cells. Even though the embryos are stored at a temperature of −197 degrees Celsius, they are not really "frozen" in the way you might imagine. They're actually in a gelatinous state, and the rapid cell division that had been occurring is now beyond the scope of slow. Within every IVF lab there are many bi-wall metal containers known as *dewars,* where cryopreserved sperm, eggs, and embryos can be stored for years at a time.

As someone who became a father through the assistance of cryopreservation, I (Mark) find it a little fantastical to imagine that my two children were cryopreserved in 2009, and while one of them was delivered in 2011 and the other was delivered in 2013, in essence, they are both exactly the same age. It is really quite remarkable how hearty human embryos are once they've formed, and that they survive this cryopreservation process. Cryopreservation technology has transformed the art of IVF laboratories, and it has also allowed us to cryopreserve human eggs, which has given the field of third-party reproduction many more options.

One of the chief benefits of using frozen eggs is the price, which is likely to be considerably lower than it is with a fresh donor. Another is the variety of donors available. At the time of this writing, many patients have difficulty finding fresh donors of certain ethnicities, while donor egg banks will typically have more options. It is also easier to move forward with treatment if you are using frozen eggs. Since the eggs have already been retrieved and cryopreserved, there is no wait for the donor to be available or to undergo a fertility cycle.

If you choose to use eggs from a fresh cycle, these donors are available to you from several sources. Donors can be someone you know, such as a relative or friend, or they can be recruited through your fertility clinic. Increasingly, people are finding their donor through an online matching service or agency. Online programs have a large pool of donors for you to choose from, whereas private agencies work almost like a concierge service to match you with a donor who has the characteristics you're looking for. These agencies can have a pool of donors from around the world. People who are looking for a specific type of donor often use agencies. For example, they might be looking for someone who is athletic, musical, smart, or attractive, or someone of a specific religion or race that is difficult to find. Online programs will charge a fee, and agencies will charge a higher fee (typically the donor will receive more compensation through the agency as well). The fees can be quite high, depending on the donor and the agency. Compensation for particular donors of certain aptitudes or ethnicities can run upward of $30,000–$50,000.

Choosing a fresh egg option is more expensive than frozen eggs, but you will typically receive a much larger batch of eggs (though there is no guarantee). Often, the donor will produce more than three to four times the number of eggs you would get from an egg bank. The egg bank splits the larger pool of eggs into small batches for sale. Since there is an attrition in fertilization, when you begin with six eggs, you may only have enough embryos for one or two embryo transfers. Therefore, if you want to have more than one child or if you are worried about not having additional embryos, it might make sense to use a donor who can provide a fresh cycle. Especially for patients who have had previous failures, it can be hard to have confidence that a single embryo will prove successful. Therefore, it can often provide a sense of relief to have additional frozen embryos for future use or as a backup plan. (A fresh egg donor is often the choice of same-sex male couples who want to be sure to have enough eggs to fertilize both partners' sperm.) If you use your clinic to find your donor, the price for one fresh donor cycle may be close to the cost of two batches of frozen eggs, but you will likely have more eggs.

As opposed to using eggs from an egg bank, using fresh donor eggs may give you the possibility of having an open relationship with your donor. This is another potential advantage of using a fresh egg donor. However, every donor is different in terms of what they will agree to. You can discuss options with your agency and your clinic. But using fresh donor eggs is the only option where that is possible. The topic of open, known, and anonymous donors is huge and important, and it is covered thoroughly in chapter 5. For now, suffice it to say that this is a factor that may be a critical part of your thinking when it comes to choosing your donor.

The rates of fresh and frozen eggs resulting in a live birth vary from clinic to clinic, but both have been improving. Ask your clinic for their success rates, or look them up on the website of the Centers for Disease Control and Prevention. Go to cdc.gov, search for "assisted reproductive technology," and click on "ART Success Rates." You can also check the American Society for Reproductive Medicine and look for the SART report to understand the success rates at your particular program. As for the health of your future child, thousands of children have been born using both fresh and frozen donor eggs, and no differences have been found in their healthy development. As the movie says, "The kids are all right."

The choice of whether to use fresh or frozen eggs is only one of the complicated, often difficult decisions you will have to make on your journey through donor conception, and many people change their minds before eventually making a final decision. To help you see what this can look like, let's look at three couples we have seen in our clinic.

AMY AND ERIC

Amy and Eric wanted one child and did not desire an open relationship with their donor, so they seemed to be good candidates for frozen eggs since one batch of frozen eggs often yields enough for one child. But they had had a long fertility journey and several losses along the way. As these losses accumulated, they began to worry about their chances of having a child at all. Amy, in particular, described her worry as "consuming." She sat in my (Lisa's) office next to Eric, dark rings under her eyes from lack of sleep, but with a look of determination on her face. She had thought this through, and she knew what she wanted to do. "If the cycle doesn't work," she said, "we'll be back to zero again. I just can't handle that." Because the idea of starting over was too upsetting to consider, they chose to undergo a fresh donor cycle, which provided them with fifteen eggs. Even though Amy and Eric had limited funds, this option felt clearly better for them. If the first cycle didn't work out, they would have, in Amy's words, "backup embryos," and that helped her feel securer in moving forward.

TODD AND ALLEN

Todd and Allen also wanted one child, but they felt strongly about having a relationship with their donor. Todd is Asian, and Allen is Caucasian. They said they preferred an Asian donor but had difficulty finding one. There were no Asian donors available through the clinic, and they did not find an Asian donor they liked through an agency. After several weeks of searching, they began to rethink their criteria. They decided that the donor's race was not as important as having a relationship with her. Once they made this decision, they had a comparatively easy time finding a donor they both were very happy with. They chose a Hispanic woman whom they felt bore a resemblance to both partners. Even better, she was willing to be open and they could have a relationship with her over the course of their lives and the life of their future child.

KERRY AND RICH

Kerry and Rich were on a tight budget. Kerry was an analyst at a small nonprofit, and Rich, a UX designer, had recently lost his job and was in the early stages of a freelance career. The insurance they had through Kerry's job was good, but it didn't cover donor conception. In addition to having limited funds to spend, they also shared a desire to have only one child, all of which made them good candidates for using an egg bank. They looked through many profiles at the egg bank, and although they had some disagreements along the way, within a few days, they had chosen a donor they felt was perfect for them. Rich said he was already imagining working at his computer at home, his baby sleeping peacefully nearby. (Good luck with that, Rich!)

As you can see, there are many variables, and many things can change when you are making this decision. Be sure to consider all your options and weigh the financial as well as emotional factors.

Retrieving Fresh Donor Eggs

If you choose a fresh egg donor, the fertility provider will need to hyperstimulate that donor's ovaries in hopes of producing ten to thirty eggs in one cycle. To understand what *hyperstimulate* means, consider that even twenty-five-year-olds, which is a common age for an egg donor, only ovulate one egg per month, even though they may start off with fifteen to thirty eggs within their ovarian follicles in a particular month. That initial number is winnowed down through the natural system of selection in which the pituitary—a gland right behind your eye—secretes an exquisitely delicate, small amount of follicle-stimulating hormone (FSH) and luteinizing hormone (LH). These hormones stimulate only one of the fifteen to thirty follicles to develop fully. Once stimulated, that follicle develops into a preovulatory follicle containing a maturing egg, which would eventually be ovulated.

Ovarian hyperstimulation will lead to the development of more than one egg in one particular month. We accomplish that by using external FSH and LH in a higher-than-normal level. Whereas the pituitary excretes a very tiny, precise balance of FSH and LH to allow only one follicle to grow, the fertility provider uses a measured amount of FSH and LH to encourage a much larger pool of eggs to develop. Some people look at their ultrasound and say their ovary looks something like a big egg crate. The dark spots, or egg containers known as follicles, contain one egg, but when the medication stimulates them, multiple follicles grow within a single ovary. And remember, most women have two ovaries. It's important to note that we are not affecting the future egg-producing potential of any particular donor. We're just harvesting the eggs that were available in that particular month.

The process of ovarian hyperstimulation starts by assessing the egg donor to make sure she's at a baseline level—that she has enough follicles that are ready to develop in that particular month. Once the donor is assessed and cleared for the process, she will be given FSH and LH. She will then return to the clinic four or five days later to have her ovaries assessed using a transvaginal ultrasound, which provides a clear view of the ovaries. Here we look at the secretion of estradiol, or human estrogen, from the growing follicles. As a follicle gets larger, it produces more estradiol, and we use that estradiol production, along with measurements of individual follicles, to determine the time to take the eggs within those follicles out of the body.

Once the follicles have matured to the size and estrogen levels where we want them, they are given a very high dose of luteinizing hormone or human chorionic gonadotropin, also known as *pregnancy hormone,* to get them ready to be fertilized by sperm. The shot is typically given into the tummy subcutaneously using a small needle and is figuratively known as the *trigger shot.* A day after receiving the trigger shot, the doctor will evaluate the hormonal changes within the donor's blood panel, and if she has the appropriate levels of hormones, we can expect to retrieve mature eggs. The day after that, your donor will be in for an egg retrieval.

The procedure for egg retrieval is called a *transvaginal oocyte aspiration.* That means your donor will have a transvaginal ultrasound placed within their vagina, and a needle will be placed through their vagina into their ovary, and then individually into each follicle to retrieve eggs. When the doctor inserts the needle into a particular follicle, a suction is applied, and the follicular fluid and the egg itself are pulled through the needle, through a thin plastic tube, and into a test tube. If somebody has twenty large follicles, the doctor performing the retrieval will go into each of those follicles individually. It can take twenty to thirty minutes, depending on the number of follicles.

This is the same procedure as the egg-extraction process we described earlier for IVF. It is a relatively easy process. The donor will be given anesthesia. There are risks to an egg retrieval, and each donor is educated on those risks, but thankfully they are low. The risk for bleeding and infection after an egg extraction process is less than one in one thousand. The bleeding risk is because we go into the ovary itself, which has blood vessels, and because behind the ovary there are some large blood vessels. Also since we go through the vagina, which is not a sterile environment, into the sterile abdominal cavity, there is a risk of infection there. Most providers give a dose of antibiotics at the time of egg retrieval to minimize the risk of infection from the procedure.

Once the eggs are retrieved, your donor will be transitioned to a recovery room to wake up. In most cases, she will be 80–90 percent recovered in about three days. In less than 5 percent of cases, donors can develop ovarian hyperstimulation syndrome, where the recovery time can stretch to seven to fourteen days and can involve significant bloating, pain, discomfort, retention of fluid, and the possible need for hospitalization. This is something their doctor will pay attention to on each cycle.

In all, a donor will have spent nine to fifteen days for ovarian hyperstimulation and egg retrieval, but it varies for each woman, and even from cycle to cycle. Typically, she is going to be on injectable medications for seven to twelve days and have four to six appointments evaluating the response before the retrieval. Over those two weeks or so, she will need to miss only about one full day of work and can otherwise go about her regular life. The medication can affect her body and her mood, but this is all also temporary—once she ceases the medication, her body will be back on its way to normal.

Just a side note. If you have been through fertility treatment, you are very familiar with the process the donor goes through, and you may associate it with a difficult emotional time. But rest assured that egg donors do not feel the same emotional challenges. Someone who has undergone fertility treatment has been coping with a lot of compounding factors, including depression, anxiety, a loss of control, a general sense of loss over what they expected their life to look like, and more. Donors typically don't have these factors when they cycle and generally don't feel the same emotional roller coaster as a woman going through IVF.

After the retrieval, the test tubes containing the follicular fluid go into the IVF laboratory, where a specialized scientist known as an embryologist looks at each tube individually under a microscope and sorts through the fluid in search of a human egg. Fascinatingly, a human egg under the microscope looks a little like a sunny-side-up egg in that it has a middle part, which represents the egg itself, and is surrounded by a mass of cells called the *cumulus*. Those cumulus cells, the jelly mass we described earlier, are making high amounts of estrogen and literally surrounding the egg itself in a high-estrogen environment.

Each egg is evaluated for its potential to be mature and receive sperm, and each of these "good" eggs is separated from the follicular fluid and put in a human tubal fluidlike media and safely stored in an incubator. At this point, pursuant to your legal agreement or consent forms with your clinic, those retrieved eggs become your "property." And hours later, they will be fertilized.

Fertilizing Eggs

There are two ways fertilization can be done in the lab. The first way is to simply expose the eggs to thousands of sperm in an incubator, which mimics fertilization in the human fallopian tube, and let nature take its course. This is the natural process. As described previously, the sperm will work their way through the jelly mass of cumulus cells that surround the egg and breach the shell, until one sperm becomes the first to reach the membrane of the egg and becomes the one to fertilize it. After setting this in motion in the incubator, we return again the next day to look for evidence of fertilization.

The second method of fertilization is intracytoplasmic sperm injection (ICSI). In this situation, we select a single sperm, break off its tail to immobilize it, and inject it directly through the membrane of the egg. This technique was originally used for men with severe male factor infertility, but in modern IVF, it has become more commonly used as a reliable method to overcome the rare case of failed fertilization, and for that reason, it's now used in 60–70 percent of IVF cases and in all cases where previously frozen eggs were used. As you can imagine, if we freeze an egg, there is the possibility of affecting the normal mechanism of fertilization, with one concern being that we might artificially harden the shell around the egg. Therefore, if you're using frozen eggs, even if there is an optimal sperm count, ICSI is used. Natural fertilization will typically only be used if both the sperm specimen and the eggs seem optimal.

ICSI is a very precise process and should only be performed by a skilled embryologist. It involves the eggs being cleaned with a solution to strip away all the cumulus cells, which can affect the viability of the egg. It also involves a highly experienced embryologist holding the egg using micromanipulation tools, choosing a single, normally shaped moving sperm, and inserting that sperm into a mature egg through an ultrasharp microscopic needle. If this all sounds somewhat amazing, it really is. And the fact that it works speaks to the resiliency of the reproductive process. By now, millions of children have been born through ICSI, and their outcomes have been studied, and these children are just as healthy and well as children born through natural conception.

So what happens in fertilization? Imagine the first moments of fertilization similar to a symphony, in that all these different processes work together in a complicated harmony to produce something beautiful. Having received the trigger shot, the egg has begun a unique process of cell division called *meiosis,* in which it goes from forty-six chromosomes to twenty-three. While it is doing this, the sperm arrives through the egg membrane. Microtubules within the egg pick up the chromosomes of the sperm and line them in sequence along with the chromosomes of the egg to make a new forty-six-chromosome embryo. An embryo at this stage, when it is just a single cell, is called a *zygote.*

When the embryologist returns to look at the egg, a zygote is what they are hoping to find. They know they have one if they see two nuclei—a sperm nucleus and egg nucleus. As you probably know, pretty much every cell in your body has one nucleus, but on day one of development of every human being, there are two nuclei.

Once the embryologist has identified that there are fertilized eggs, these zygotes are sorted out and placed in a solution that supports the early development of embryos. Initially, the fuel source for embryos is very small proteins, and eventually, it involves basic sugars or carbohydrates, which most cells use for fuel. Over the next five to seven days, this one-cell zygote divides fifty to sixty times, going from one cell to two cells to four to eight to sixteen to thirty-two, continuing up to somewhere between two hundred and five hundred cells, to become a *blastocyst,* that daisy we described, with the cells that will become the fetus in the center and the cells that will become the placenta surrounding them.

We used to look at embryos every day to check their development, but what we've learned over the years is that the less we take them out of the incubator, the better they do. You may want to hear updates every day, but many labs only give an update at the blastocyst stage, which is five days after development. At that stage, the embryo is hardier and more resilient.

Blastocysts develop in the laboratory on a continuum over developmental days five, six, and seven. They are also assessed for their stage (still in their shell, hatching from the shell, or hatched). Yes, human embryos hatch from a shell. They are also graded on their cellularity. More cellular embryos are graded higher and have higher reproductive potential. As we discussed, the blastocyst has two major areas of cells: the trophectoderm (the part of the blastocyst that makes the placenta) and the inner cell mass (the part of the blastocyst that makes the fetus). These two areas are scored independently based on their cellularity. These three features, the number of days taken to develop into a blastocyst, the cellularity of the trophectoderm, and the inner cell mass, are combined to assign a reproductive potential for any particular embryo. Grading of embryos for transfer into the uterus or cryopreservation is commonly on a grade 1, 2, or 3 basis and is mostly focused on the inner cell mass and trophectoderm grades. A grade 1 embryo has a two-layer trophectoderm cell layer and a dense inner cell mass.

It's important to be aware that there is some attrition on the journey from egg to zygote to blastocyst. For example, if twenty eggs are retrieved, we'd expect sixteen to be mature, twelve to be fertilized, and about six blastocysts to form. Your doctor will select the single best embryo for transfer to your uterus.

PREIMPLANTATION GENETIC TESTING FOR ANEUPLOIDY

You may have the option to test your embryos through a process called *preimplantation genetic testing for aneuploidy* (PGT-A). This is something you will discuss with your doctor. PGT-A will determine if the embryo has a normal number of chromosomes. More than 99 percent of human beings have forty-six chromosomes, but some have forty-five or forty-seven. In some cases, these people may have developmental abnormalities or other medical problems. Moving forward with PGT-A is a way to exclude embryos that do not have forty-six chromosomes from potential transfer into the uterine cavity. The process involves taking five to ten of the trophectoderm or implantation cells off the embryo—the equivalent of plucking petals off the daisy—and submitting those cells for chromosomal analysis. Choosing to pursue PGT-A runs a 1–3 percent chance of harming an embryo secondary to the biopsy process. Because 20–30 percent of donated egg embryos are chromosomally abnormal, many parents do choose to take the risk by testing their embryos. It is important to note that there is an error rate in diagnosing embryos as normal, which varies depending on technique, but it is greater than 99 percent accurate using the most modern techniques.

Transferring the Embryo

If you are the patient receiving the embryo, you will have been taking estrogen, a steroid hormone, for ten to twenty days to lead to the development of a receptive uterine lining, and in some cases to sync your cycle with that of the donor, or perhaps your doctor has chosen to do this in your natural cycle. The endometrial lining is a very unique space within the uterus that is typically less than one centimeter thick and represents the anterior and posterior wall of the endometrial cavity. It is the "magical" cellular layer or "soil" that provides a location and nutrients for a human embryo to begin the implantation process and continue its development. Once your endometrial lining is of the appropriate thickness and has an appropriate ultrasound appearance, it will be exposed to progesterone, another steroid hormone like estrogen that stimulates the uterus to prepare it for the arrival of the embryo and pregnancy, either through ovulation (if you're on your own cycle) or an external injection. The progesterone shot can be uncomfortable, but there are many tricks that can help ease the discomfort, such as icing the area before injection, massaging the area afterward, and using a heating pad afterward, all of which you can discuss with your nurse.

Finally, you will arrive at your fertility clinic for the embryo transfer. Similar to an insemination, an embryo transfer is something like a fancy Pap smear. A speculum is placed in the vagina, which allows your doctor to see the cervix, and then an ultrasound probe is placed on the abdomen, allowing them to see the uterine cavity through the abdomen. Your doctor will then pass the small tube that contains your embryo through the cervix to the upper part of your uterus, and release the embryo. An embryo transfer is usually scheduled for twenty to thirty minutes, though the actual embryo transfer usually takes less than five minutes.

The moment when an embryo is transferred is very special and one that I (Mark) have had the privilege and honor to participate in thousands of times. For many, it's the first time they've had the opportunity to be pregnant. For most, it represents the culmination of months and sometimes years of work. Many patients feel very emotional during this procedure, saying it was a moment filled with hope of a family-to-be. If both parents-to-be can be present for the embryo transfer, it can feel even more special.

While the moment the embryo is placed in the uterus is surely special, there's also a sense of, "What do I do now?" The short answer to that question is: nothing. That might sound strange or even difficult after all the hard work you and your team have done—retrieving the eggs, fertilizing them, culturing the embryos in the IVF laboratory, and finally depositing that one most cellular embryo into your uterine cavity. But now, it is a natural process. This embryo needs to fully hatch out of its shell, stick to your endometrial lining, and further expand and grow to successfully implant and become an early pregnancy.

All that can mean that the day of your transfer is a day

not only of great hope but also sometimes great anxiety, because now you have nine to ten days of waiting for a positive pregnancy test. And there's no doubt, that is a long wait. Just like a patient who has received insemination, you will likely feel a lot of mixed emotions during that waiting period, but there's literally nothing you can do but self-nurture, be hopeful, and wait for a blood test. Some patients do take an early urine pregnancy test, but we do not recommend that because that test can sometimes give a false sense of hope. Even if a urine pregnancy test gives a positive result, it doesn't provide the same breadth of information as a blood pregnancy test with a numerical result.

As you journey through the donor-egg process, understand the culmination of your work is getting to embryo transfer, and then you have this moment of waiting for your pregnancy test result, which we all hope is positive. We mention to all our patients that your entire team wants you to be pregnant. You have a whole team of fertility professionals who all want the same thing. As long as we have worked in fertility—and we've done it a long time—we still get excited for our patients who are positive, and we become very sad if they are not.

Using Donated Embryos

Let's go back for a moment to that day of embryo transfer. Recall that the patient may have two or more blastocysts available, and they will only transfer one—or at least one at a time. Those that are not transferred are kept in cryo-preservation.

At some point, though, the patient has to decide what to do with their unused embryos. They can use another one to have another child. They can use several more to have additional children, but if they don't intend to use all six or seven embryos, and most people don't, then there will be some that are left over. The parent can have them disposed of, they can donate them to science, or they can donate them to an independent program that will then make them available to a new patient who wants to build a family.

This decision can be very difficult for parents, and we talk more about that—and offer guidance on making that decision—later in the book. The upshot for our purposes here, though, is that someone who wants to build a family with donor conception has the option to use donated embryos. It can be a less expensive option for patients as well, because the donor has already paid for the costs associated with creating the embryos.

The Big Picture

After you have chosen your donor, the entire process of embryo creation will take three to four weeks. The process of preparing the uterus for embryo transfer also takes three to four weeks. These can be done in concert or, if you're using previously frozen embryos, at a separate interval. If you're using donor eggs, your donor will be spending about that same amount of time having her ovaries hyperstimulated with follicle-stimulating hormone (FSH) and luteinizing hormone (LH) to produce as many eggs as possible. The embryo transfer or implantation is followed by an anxious week or two of waiting before you will take a pregnancy test.

On average, patients using donor sperm for insemination will become pregnant 15–20 percent of the time, depending on the age of the patient. Patients using fresh donor eggs will have a 50–60 percent success rate, and for patients using frozen eggs, the rate will be 40–50 percent. If you're using donated frozen embryos, your odds are 20–50 percent depending on their own embryological grade and age of the egg source. If you need to try again, you will wait four to six weeks to allow your uterus to shed the lining and then to grow it again.

Remember that these are averages and that every patient is different. Following the advice in chapter 3, "Preparing for Pregnancy," will greatly improve your chances. Sometimes it does take multiple attempts. This can be dispiriting, but you have already shown great strength and perseverance in getting this far. Together with your fertility team, your partner if you have one, and your personal support network, you can do it.

KEY TERMS

blastocyst: an embryo that has undergone the first major stage of differentiation of cells; it now has an inner group of cells, which will develop into the fetus, and an outer group of cells, which will develop into the placenta

cumulus cells: a cluster of cells that surrounds an egg that produced high levels of estrogen and contains signals to induce that egg to mature and prepare for fertilization

embryologist: a scientist who is an expert in the fertility field and works with sperm, eggs, embryos, and the many machines and techniques necessary to allow for success in the IVF laboratory

estradiol: human estrogen, a steroid hormone secreted by follicles within the human ovary, which leads to the healthy development of the egg and a healthy development of the endometrial lining

follicle-stimulating hormone (FSH) and luteinizing hormone (LH): hormones secreted by the anterior pituitary that stimulate ovarian follicles so that they mature human eggs; they are also the hormones responsible for the development of human sperm in the secretion of testosterone in men

intracytoplasmic sperm injection (ICSI): a technique in which a single sperm is injected directly through the membrane of an egg

meiosis: cell division in which eggs and sperm go from forty-six chromosomes to twenty-three in preparation for their combination to create a human embryo

ovarian follicle: small, fluid-filled sacs in the ovaries that each contain an unfertilized egg

progesterone: a steroid hormone that stimulates the endometrial lining to prepare for the arrival and subsequent implantation of a human embryo; it is secreted by the ovary from the same follicle that has ovulated

transvaginal oocyte aspiration: the medical procedure of retrieving mature eggs from the ovary; the doctor uses a needle that is individually placed into each follicle and then uses suction to pull out the follicular fluid; the human egg contained in the follicle travels along with this fluid and is collected by the laboratory

trigger shot: a shot that contains luteinizing hormone or human chorionic gonadotropin, or "pregnancy hormone," which is given to you or the egg donor to induce their eggs to go through the final maturation step prior to an egg retrieval; it is typically given thirty-five to thirty-seven hours before the egg retrieval

trophectoderm cells: the outer cells of a blastocyst that will become the placenta

zygote: the first stage of an embryo, when it is made up of only one cell

3

Preparing for Pregnancy

I f you choose to use donated gametes, it goes without saying that someone on your team should be pregnant, whether it's your gestational carrier, your partner, or yourself using donated eggs or sperm. It should also go without saying that carrying a pregnancy puts a tremendous amount of stress on the body. In fact, if you think about everything people with a uterus go through to give birth, it's really quite amazing that it is possible. So, preparing for pregnancy by optimizing your health in key areas is very important. Doing so can not only help make pregnancy easier for you, but importantly, it can have very real health implications for your child.

Our behavior, our environment, and our health all affect how our genes work. Think of it this way: Each of us has fifty-two thousand genes, but only about 50 percent are "turned on" or expressed at any one time. Factors like stress or being overweight can change which genes are expressed. You may be fascinated to realize that each cell has about six feet of DNA within it, yet the majority of that DNA does not code for genes themselves but allows for the organization of those genes to be expressed.

The influence of outside factors on gene expression is known as *epigenetics*. Epigenetics is a wonderful thing to think about with regard to how you live your life and maximize your health. An obvious example is the negative effects of cigarette smoking. The ongoing damage by chemicals in cigarette smoke turns on a series of genes that eventually leads to cells growing out of control, and eventually lung cancer. For a more positive example of epigenetics, someone who is at significant risk for diabetes, and therefore heart attack and stroke, can exercise regularly, limit their sugar intake, and thereby modify their inherited risk based on how they live their lives.

If you are preparing to be pregnant or are pregnant, it is important to understand that epigenetic changes don't only happen to you. They will actually change the code within the fetus's development, so being stressed or overweight—or smoking, drinking, or having a diet insufficient in vitamins, or any number of other negative factors—can cause long-term health risks for the child. The good news is that epigenetic changes do not change a person's DNA sequence; rather, they change how the DNA sequence is read by the body. In other words, they are modifiable. Not only that, you can make positive changes for your future child, and yourself, starting now.

Fascinatingly, epigenetics can be influenced by the person carrying the pregnancy even if they are not genetically linked to the unborn child. This can be comforting to fertility patients who struggle with the grief of not being the person who donates their genetics to their child-to-be—that is, women who use donated eggs to build their family. The fact is that they *are* linked to their child genetically in that all throughout pregnancy, they are the managers of gene expression and affecting the future health and gene expression in their child.

Epigenetics may even go beyond health to personality. We all know families in which the children have widely different personalities. Perhaps our personalities relate back to how our mothers felt when they were carrying us, and what went on in their lives, and what we were exposed to in utero. It's something significant to consider as you prepare for pregnancy—preparing your body, mind, and lifestyle to put yourself and your unborn child in the best possible situation.

One more thing to consider is the effect of epigenetic changes on bringing a pregnancy to term. Women who are smokers or obese have higher miscarriage rates. Women with significant hyper- and hypothyroidism as well as uncontrolled diabetes have more risk for pregnancy complications, miscarriage, and birth defects.

Thankfully, you can stack the odds in your favor and in

favor of your unborn child. This chapter discusses the most important things you can do to prepare for pregnancy.

Weight Management and Exercise

Working toward your healthiest weight can make a dramatic difference. A general rule of thumb is to strive for a body mass index, which is a combination of height and weight, in the normal range (20–24.9). According to the American College of Obstetricians and Gynecologists, outcomes for the children and the person carrying the baby are statistically worse for women with a BMI of greater than 30. That being said, we all are aware healthy babies can be born from women who are overweight and underweight. Even so, epigenetic data suggests that children born from women who are not their optimal weight, or in very stressful situations, may have long-term health implications later in life.

To be sure, BMI is not a perfect gauge of obesity and health. It does not take into account other factors, such as waist size, muscle mass, or how much fat is present in the body. People who are fit, with strong muscles and little fat, will have a higher BMI compared to someone of the same height, because muscle weighs more than fat. BMI is a useful starting point for assessing weight, but it's important to discuss your weight with your doctor and consider modifying your diet or making lifestyle changes to maximize your chance for a successful pregnancy and delivery.

Your doctor can also help you make a plan for bringing down your weight to a healthier level if you are overweight. Of course, it all begins with diet, and many people can make the necessary changes simply through common sense. Avoid processed and high-fat foods, and control portions so that you are eating an appropriate number of calories a day. It also helps to establish a regular eating schedule, so you're having meals and snacks at the same time each day. Again, your doctor, or a dietary professional, can help create an individualized approach that is right for you. (The next section in this chapter provides information about eating a healthy diet.)

The other piece of the puzzle is movement. Integrating a daily (or at least three to four times a week) exercise regimen that includes strength training will prepare the body for the massive changes that go along in pregnancy. If you're like most of us, you may be sitting for most of your day. Can you set your alarm to take a short walk outside a couple of times a day? Or do some safe yoga poses or movements at lunch? You can even put on some music and dance to your favorite song. Standing desks have become popular because it is so important to reduce the many hours we are sitting in our day. We both cherish ours!

If getting into an exercise routine is new or challenging for you, see if you can get a buddy or partner to embark on these changes with you. Can you take walks with your partner or a friend? Can you take some calls with your friends and family members while you walk outside or on the treadmill? Can you do strength training in a group? You will be less likely to cancel on someone else than you would on yourself, so having a partner to be accountable to can make all the difference in your consistency. Consistency will eventually create a habit, and a positive habit is what you want.

While diet has a much greater effect on weight than exercise, exercise provides other critical benefits. Consider that in pregnancy, someone will gain twenty-five pounds over nine months, pounds that are focused in the abdomen and that strain the lower back and abdominal muscles. This added weight also affects their ability to breathe and the way their pelvis and hips work. Therefore, preparing for pregnancy by improving flexibility and strength training is essential for your tolerance of that physical burden. And once again, how you feel in pregnancy may relate to outcomes for your child.

Eating Habits and Vitamins

Most of us know what we should eat, even if we don't always eat as well as we should. The basics of a healthy diet include minimizing meats and processed foods, and having a balanced diet of complex carbohydrates and fruits and vegetables of many colors. Leafy greens are most important. Reduce refined sugar, and drink lots of water. Water is so important, and few people drink enough of it. Meeting with a nutritionist or dietician who specializes in pregnancy can help you plan for changes that are doable and effective.

Certainly, this is an ideal way to eat when you're pregnant, and most pregnant people are naturally highly motivated to do so, but we recommend eating that way for two to three months before your pregnancy. That helps prepare your body and also helps you get in the habit so it's easy to continue when you are pregnant. We're not saying you have to be totally rigid about what you eat and drink, denying yourself even a single french fry for all those months and drinking kale smoothies by the gallon. Rather, be conscious and deliberate about what you eat. Use common sense, and think about that baby whose life you are going to create. You will make better choices, and you will feel good about it. We see many people stress about everything they do. The guidelines in this section are ideal, but if you are at a family lunch and you want to splurge, enjoy it! Yes. If you feel nauseous and live on crackers for a while, is that okay? Yes. Early in the pregnancy the nutritional requirements for your little blueberry or kidney bean are minimal. One of the worst things you can ingest is self-criticism. Women especially can be so hard on themselves. Do the best you can, and if you want hot dogs and Cracker Jacks at a ball game, do it and enjoy yourself. Growth is not linear, and habits are hard to break. Remember that, and be kind to yourself.

Beyond those basic healthy diet choices, you will want to enhance your diet with certain vitamins to give your body the resources it needs prepregnancy and in pregnancy. If you're not including enough vitamins in your diet, your body will actually drain resources from yourself and divert them to the fetus. There are three major classes of vitamins that are essential for your well-being and the health of the future pregnancy.

We'll start with folic acid, a B vitamin that supports cell division, or the creation of new cells. When an embryo starts out, it is made up of about 150 cells and is one hundred times smaller than a printed period. Growing that embryo into an eight-pound baby requires cells to divide millions upon millions of times, so you can see why getting lots of folic acid and other B vitamins is essential. It is particularly essential preconception because the very early part of the pregnancy is when a dramatic amount of cell division is happening.

The importance of folic acid is best shown by looking at the development of the neural tube, a hollow structure in the embryo that eventually forms the brain and spinal cord. Very early on, even in an embryo that is smaller than one centimeter, we can see the start of the spinal column. There are classic studies that show that women who are folic-acid deficient have an increased risk of neural tube defects such as spina bifida, which is basically a hole in the back of the spine.[1]

What this means is, if you're planning on carrying a pregnancy, you'll want to start getting at least 400 micrograms (mcg) of folic acid every day, ideally starting two to three months prior to pregnancy. And if you're planning on using a gestational carrier, it can be helpful for her to understand this, too, before her embryo transfer. You can get folic acid both through your diet, in enriched foods such as certain cereals and breads, and by supplementing with B vitamins. Most women's vitamins have the recommended daily amount of folic acid.

Now let's talk about iron. Embryos and fetuses have the massive job of growing red blood cells and muscle. It's fascinating to see that at about nine weeks of pregnancy, when the embryo is only one to two inches in length, it actually moves a little bit. This is normal and yet incredible. The fetus needs iron as an essential mineral to help red blood cells develop, which oxygenate their tissues, and if a pregnant person is anemic in pregnancy—that is, if they are iron deficient—they can't provide optimal oxygenation to the placenta, the organ that nourishes the fetus. That can lead to growth restriction, or a smaller-than-expected child.

To understand just how important iron is, and how much is needed, consider that a woman who is not pregnant is recommended to take 18 milligrams (mg) of iron supplements a day. People with a monthly menstrual cycle lose blood, and iron is required to grow new red blood cells to replenish the ones lost during a menstrual flow. When they are pregnant, and thus not having menstrual cycles—in other words, not losing blood—the recommended dose is nevertheless even higher: 27 milligrams. That's a 30 percent increase for iron supplementation preconception and during pregnancy to support muscle and red blood cell development in the growing fetus.

The third important vitamin is calcium, and it is hard to get enough of it. We may not always think of getting calcium, because as adults our bones are already grown and calcified. But growing and calcifying the fetus's bones is essential early in a pregnancy. In addition, women are increasingly at risk for osteoporosis, the premature weakening of the bones, as they age. And each pregnancy puts them more at risk: If you don't have enough calcium in your diet when you're pregnant, your body steals it from your bones to provide to the embryo and fetus.

In general, it's recommended that you get 1,500–2,000 milligrams of calcium prepregnancy and during pregnancy. Calcium sources include dairy products and dark green leafy veggies. Interestingly, many pregnant people take Tums during pregnancy for heartburn, and while heartburn is no fun, a silver lining is that Tums are a good source of calcium.

To reiterate, it is ideal to eat as if you are pregnant starting two to three months *before* getting pregnant, which means aiming for at least 400 micrograms of folic acid in a daily supplement in addition to 27 milligrams of iron and 1,500–2,000 milligrams of calcium.

There is some newer data on supplements in pregnancy, which include choline and omega-3 fatty acids. Those are a little beyond the scope for someone getting ready to get pregnant, but your ob-gyn might recommend them once you get pregnant.

Avoiding Toxins

We all know that alcohol during pregnancy can lead to fetal alcohol syndrome (FAS). But it's also been reported in infertility patients that drinking alcohol at a level of greater than five drinks per week prepregnancy can affect fertility, conception, and miscarriage.[2]

So, as you prepare for pregnancy, either for yourself or your surrogate, it's important to be drinking fewer than five drinks a week, and obviously once you have an embryo transfer, you should be drinking no alcohol at all. You can find different doctors who have different opinions on this, and you will find people who say they drank throughout their pregnancy, but for everything you're going through to bring this child to life, why take that risk? Simply avoid alcohol and never look back.

Remember our earlier discussion about epigenetics, and how environment and behavior can "turn on" certain genes and affect changes in ourselves and our unborn child? The toxic effects of alcohol are a reason for birth defects; therefore, consider that alcohol is affecting the gene expression that leads to the unique facial features associated with FAS.

Similar to drinking alcohol, we don't think anyone needs to be told not to smoke during pregnancy. But as with drinking, smoking prepregnancy can also lead to poorer outcomes. If you are someone who smokes, please seek assistance from your physicians and trusted medical providers. Using any form of nicotine replacement if you're unable to quit is certainly safer than continuing to inhale superheated gas that contains tar and nicotine and a thousand other dangerous compounds.

There are significant concerns about other toxins we absorb. These include endocrine disruptors in makeup, chemicals in hair dye, and hormone disruptors contained in plastics, in particular bisphenol A (BPA). There is a significant body of literature about environmental toxins that is beyond the scope of this book, but it is important to understand that in the first trimester, the embryo is literally creating the major organs of the future fetus. Over the first thirteen weeks of pregnancy, we recommend that all patients eat and live the healthiest, most natural lifestyle possible. There are many unknowns, and controlling the outside substances and chemicals that enter into a pregnant person's body can affect the health and well-being of the future child.

On a similar note, you will also want to avoid any recreational drugs during pregnancy as well as before conception. If you need help with drug use, please get it. There are many options, including talking to your doctor or calling the Substance Abuse and Mental Health Services Administration help line at 1-800-662-HELP (4357).

Medications

Do you take an antidepressant or antianxiety medication? Easily 20–30 percent of the women we see in our work do. And while the vast majority of these medications are associated with minimal risk in pregnancy, we still suggest that they stop taking them if they can. If you are in one of these patient groups, we urge you to consider regular therapy sessions, such as talk therapy and cognitive behavioral therapy, with the goal of coming off these medications, or at least minimizing them. And if you're not able to wean off your medication, speak with a psychiatrist who can advise you about the medications that may be best to use during pregnancy. Whatever you do, please don't simply stop taking your medication without talking to your prescribing doctor about making a safe change.

Some people move toward Eastern medicine, including acupuncture or pregnancy-specific yoga, to manage their brain chemistry. If you go this route, be sure you do not use any supplements that are not approved for pregnancy. Many herbs and "natural medicines" can have effects on the fetus that we don't know about. Use caution, and make sure to run everything by your doctor to ensure you're doing all you can to have a safe and healthy pregnancy.

It's important to remember that not only do you want to get pregnant and have a baby, that baby is going to eventually grow up to be a young person and an adult, and there's so much we don't know about human development. Decades ago, some doctors would encourage women to have a cigarette to combat nausea during pregnancy or have a drink to relax. Fortunately, we now know better. So, while there is only so much we can do, there is still a lot you can do to give your child a great start.

If you do need to be on medication in pregnancy, a class of subspecialists in OB-GYN called *maternal fetal medicine specialists* are specially trained in caring for pregnant women and represent the medical treatment arm for pregnant women, and they will meet with you, prepregnancy, to assess the medications you're on and the risk in pregnancy.

This might apply to women who are on high blood pressure medication, perhaps diabetes medication, or medication for seizures, autoimmune diseases, migraines, anxiety, and depression. If you have concerns about your prepregnancy medication usage, your ob-gyn is a great resource, but accessing other subspecialists as far as prepregnancy recommendations can help you tremendously in feeling good and ready for pregnancy.

ACUPUNCTURE

Many patients ask about acupuncture in preparation for embryo transfer and pregnancy. Acupuncture is a fascinating traditional Chinese medical practice in which thin needles are inserted into the skin at strategic points on the body to treat pain and overall wellness. Traditional Chinese practitioners say that the practice rebalances your qi, or energy. We are electrical creatures. Everything in your body, from your brain to your heart to your little finger, requires electricity, so adjusting—and understanding better—the way electricity flows through the body can be a way to modulate different aspects of our well-being. If you're somebody who leans toward Eastern medicine, getting acupuncture for pain and stress relief and relaxation can be very helpful. Also, numerous studies suggest acupuncture may enhance your chances of successfully conceiving through insemination or embryo transfer.

One caveat is to be sure you find a qualified, experienced acupuncturist. In the United States, acupuncturists can be certified and licensed. Acupuncture is truly an art and requires an acupuncturist with experience working with infertility patients, and you should choose this based on credentials as well as referrals from your physician.

Uterine and Fallopian Tube Health

So far, we've discussed things that someone can do on their own to prepare to carry a pregnancy. It's also essential that your doctor assesses the health and structure of your uterus and fallopian tubes to make sure they are ready to receive an embryo formed from donated eggs or for conception through donor sperm.

The human embryo implants in the uterus. When a person is still a developing fetus, the uterus forms as two halves that migrate to the pelvis and merge in the middle, and then the middle portion is absorbed into an organ that is shaped like a pear. And the embryo grows and stretches the larger part of the pear. In my (Mark's) fertility practice, we find that about 15 percent of people with a uterus have anatomical issues within their uterus that can affect their ability to achieve or sustain a pregnancy. These include polyps, which are overgrowths of glandular tissue. Polyps have a very low likelihood for cancer, but they are areas that are not receptive for an embryo to grow and develop—they are not a "soft landing spot."

Another common overgrowth of normal tissue is leiomyomata, also known as a *fibroid* or *benign tumor.* Many people are quite surprised to realize that 35–40 percent of women have fibroids. And as they age, they're more likely to have fibroids that may affect pregnancy. One of the things I say to my patients is that, similar to real estate, "location matters." Fibroids can be outside the uterus, in the wall of the uterus, in the cervix, pushing into the uterine cavity, or perhaps within the uterine cavity. Fibroids that are pushing into the uterine cavity or within the uterine cavity have a significant effect on pregnancy success. Fibroids that are outside the cavity that are greater than five centimeters can also be a significant issue.

The evaluation for fibroids includes a transvaginal ultrasound, which uses sound waves to look carefully at the muscle structure of the uterus and the glandular structure of the endometrium (the glandular membrane lining the uterus). A simple transvaginal ultrasound can evaluate whether fibroids are present and whether the uterus is normally shaped. To evaluate for polyps, the internal shape of the uterus, and the location of fibroids, a special ultrasound known as a *saline ultrasound* is used. In this procedure, a saline solution is introduced into the uterine cavity, which pushes the wall of the uterus apart. A saline ultrasound also can help identify fibroids that have pushed into the cavity or are in the cavity, which can also have a dramatic negative effect on a potential pregnancy.

Another way to think of a saline sonogram is that it's kind of like when you go to the dentist and they ask you to open your mouth so they can look at what's inside. Here we use the saline to separate the walls of the uterine cavity to look inside and see if there are any polyps or fibroids. This procedure is about as uncomfortable as it sounds, but it's usually tolerable and thankfully relatively quick. We recommend that women consider talking to their doctor about taking a pain reliever prior to the study.

We also check for scar tissue, which, like polyps and fibroids, can represent areas that are not receptive to an embryo. What makes scar tissue form within the uterine cavity is not always known, but it's usually associated with an unsuccessful pregnancy that ended in miscarriage or perhaps a previous surgery in the uterus or an abortion. Rarely, we go to put the saline in the cavity and the cavity doesn't expand at all, which indicates significant scar tissue that has stuck the walls of the uterus together, creating a barrier to carrying a pregnancy. Thankfully, the vast majority of scar tissue that we do see in the uterus is of the less important variety.

Minor scar tissue, fibroids, and polyps can all be corrected through a surgery called *hysteroscopy*. If you do have abnormalities in your uterine cavity, your doctor or a specialist can place a telescope within the uterine cavity and remove the scar tissue, polyp, or fibroid. This can frequently be completed with one surgery, but sometimes the fibroid, polyp, or scar tissue can't be removed in one sitting, so a second or third surgery is needed. The good news is that the vast majority of uterine cavity abnormalities can be surgically corrected to make someone's uterus receptive to an embryo that either arrives from their fallopian tube after donor sperm insemination or is placed in the uterus during the embryo transfer.

For people conceiving through donor sperm insemination and women conceiving through an embryo transfer, it's important to have fallopian tubes that haven't been previously damaged. Damage to fallopian tubes could occur as a result of previous appendicitis, previous abdominal surgery, congenital abnormalities (birth defects), or a history of sexually transmitted infections.

To check the fallopian tubes, we use a test called *hysterosalpingogram* (HSG), or a tubal dye study. In an HSG, we inject the fallopian tubes with a dye that can be seen on x-ray, which allows us to evaluate the fallopian tubes. The HSG usually takes about fifteen minutes, but unfortunately, it can cause some significant cramping and discomfort. What are we looking for? We are checking to see if the fallopian tubes are normal caliber, open at their distal end near the ovary (i.e., not blocked), and, most important, not dilated, or enlarged.

If your fallopian tubes are blocked, that might be an indication to move directly to in vitro fertilization and embryo transfer. This is important for people moving forward with donor sperm insemination. A dilated fallopian tube means that it has been damaged and is collecting fluid. The fallopian tube is a glandular structure on the inside and is always secreting fluid, but if the fallopian tube is dilated, the normal mechanisms for reabsorbing and clearing that fluid are not in place. The result is that fluid collects in the fallopian tube, which can affect the ability of sperm to swim to the egg and the ability of the embryo to travel down the fallopian tube to the uterus. And after the embryo transfer, that fluid could leak into the uterine cavity, negatively affecting implantation, perhaps by the mechanical aspect of fluid washing through the cavity. What's more, the components contained within that fluid are not supposed to be in the uterine cavity, and they can affect gene expression and thereby negatively affect a successful implantation. For patients who are transferring an embryo into the uterus, it might seem confusing that the state of the fallopian tubes is important, but for all these reasons, if you have a dilated fallopian tube that potentially is leaking fluid into the uterine cavity, it needs to be removed or closed up.

If you complete your HSG and your fallopian tubes are normal and open, that's a green light to move forward with insemination. If, on the other hand, you need to have your fallopian tube operated on, that requires a surgery called *laparoscopy*. This surgery involves placing a telescope into your abdominal cavity, evaluating your fallopian tubes, ovaries, and other pelvic structures, and either correcting or removing the damaged structures.

Let's take a moment to consider the amazing role of the uterus in human reproduction. From the time menstrual age hits at twelve or thirteen, up until about age fifty, every month, the uterus grows an endometrial lining, makes that lining receptive to an embryo, and, if pregnancy does not occur, sheds that lining down to its base, only to do that again the following month. That cycle of endometrial development and shedding is essential to having a healthy uterine cavity to place an embryo in. People who do not have regular menstrual cycles may need to use medication to encourage their body to create a cycle to prepare their uterus for a successful implantation. People who do not have periods due to premature ovarian failure or menopause may need their uterus treated for a few months prior to receiving the embryo to have their endometrial lining prepared to receive an embryo.

As you seek out your care provider in preparation for pregnancy, I (Mark) think it's important we all understand that medicine is heading in the way of personalization. In my more than thirty years of being a doctor, I am constantly impressed by the diversity in our humanity and how people's anatomy can differ on the inside compared to the way it is on the outside. People can look perfectly healthy but have problems on the inside. We need to know everything on the inside is within the range of normal so you don't invest time, emotion, and dollars when conditions are not optimal for a successful pregnancy.

Protecting Sperm and Eggs

In many donor-conception pairings, we're using either the sperm of the intended father or the eggs of the intended mother in the equation. Let's talk about how to protect them.

In regard to sperm, thankfully, men make millions every day. The reality is that the vast majority of those sperm are either not moving or not a normal shape, and therefore not viable, but because it's such a massive production line, there are usually plenty that are viable. But sperm *can* be affected by stress, smoking, lifestyle choices like spending too much time in hot tubs and saunas, or being overweight, which can alter the internal genetic code within a sperm and affect the future health and well-being of the child. We also know that men who conceive after age sixty (and younger for some men) will have children who have more risk for particular birth defects that are unique to advancing paternal age. We recommend men have genetic counseling to better understand the effects of paternal age on the health and well-being of a future child. We don't really understand what changes in sperm as we age, but it is important for intended fathers to understand that many lifestyle decisions—things like smoking, alcohol consumption, weight management, and exercise—all come into play in terms of sperm quality and likely sperm function in the health and well-being of your yet-to-be child.

Regarding alcohol specifically, studies show that heavy drinking in men is consistently associated with decreased sperm quality, including occasionally azoospermia, or the absence of viable sperm in semen. Findings are less consistent for women, but studies indicate that even moderate consumption may affect their ability to conceive. We encourage all fathers-to-be and mothers-to-be to minimize alcohol consumption.

It's also smart to be wary of environmental toxins, so if you're somebody who regularly works in gardens with herbicides and pesticides, that's something to be conscious of because those chemicals also affect sperm function. Mercury is another one to look out for. There's some classic information on men who eat tuna fish every day for lunch that shows that the mercury levels not only affect their overall health but also affect their sperm quality and ability to fertilize eggs and make healthy embryos. Clearly, it makes sense to severely limit or eliminate tuna fish from your diet.

All that said, it is important to understand that sperm is probably about 20 percent of the equation. Sperm is like the key to your car. Your car does all these amazing things—drives, plays music, perhaps heats your seat, and so on—but you can't go anywhere without the car key. While sperm is the car key, the egg is really the vehicle of generating a new human life. And the fact is that women are born with a fixed number of eggs, and that egg pool decreases in number and quality as women age.

Women have five distinct parts of their life: childhood, puberty, reproductive, perimenopausal, and menopausal. Reproductive age range is from about sixteen to forty-five, but that range can be negatively affected by lifestyle choices like drinking, smoking, and exposure to toxins. So it's important for mothers-to-be to recognize that they have to practice healthy lifestyle choices as they move toward pregnancy—and really, for optimal results, all throughout the reproductive part of their life to protect their egg pool. Furthermore, it is important to acknowledge that in spite of even the best lifestyle, egg quality begins to decline sometime after age thirty-five in all women, affecting their ability to conceive. Age is the single greatest predictor of fertility in women.

Some people's eggs are naturally more resilient than others'. But reproductive aging is the whole reason this field of egg donation exists. One of the most common patient populations we see are people who have passed the age thirty-five mark, and whose egg pool is decreased in quality and/or quantity to the point where they are having problems getting pregnant without any help. One of the main reasons they seek help is their egg quality or quantity has dropped, and achieving natural conception using their own eggs is much less likely than when they were twenty-five.

Professionals like us, and resources like this book, are necessary to move forward with donor conception, but as you can see, there is much that you can and should do on your own to improve the process. Preparing your body for pregnancy or even preparing to be an egg or sperm source for your partner represents a commitment to your health, the health of your gametes, the health of your uterus, and the future health of your child-to-be.

Part II

Choosing Your Donor

4

Medical Considerations

Choosing your egg or sperm donor is the most critical and permanent choice you will make on your journey through donor conception. You may have a lot of ideas going into the process about what is important to you in a donor, and you may have a huge amount of information at your disposal. If you have a partner, you have to navigate to a decision that is satisfying for both of you. Yes, it *is* a big, complicated decision, and yes, it can be overwhelming. But you can make it with confidence.

This chapter describes the most important medical aspects to consider when looking at donors. It lays out the basic factors that relate to the future health and well-being of your child-to-be. Think of evaluating medical considerations as a first step toward making your decision. The following chapters provide further steps, and chapter 7 pulls it all together and provides a helpful step-by-step process for working your way through all these considerations to your final decision.

Who will be the donor who helps create your future child? We'll begin by looking into the past.

Examine Family History

While on its face it might seem like you'd want to make a good physical match, someone whose appearance is appealing to you or who checks off certain aesthetic boxes, it's important to understand that when the goal is having a healthy child, other factors are much more important. Family history and genetics are the most important components in choosing a donor because these can help reduce health risks for your future child. The more information you can have on your donor's parents, grandparents, and siblings, the better you can predict the health and well-being of your child.

Humans are made up of a unique combination of fifty-two thousand genes, and your donor, whether sperm or egg, will be providing twenty-six thousand of them to your child. These twenty-six thousand genes represent health traits and features of the donor's past generations and are distributed somewhat randomly from her paternal and maternal family trees. We've learned a lot about genetics in the last thirty years since the DNA code has been unraveled, and we continue to learn more and more.

There are certain things that we understand better than

others. For example, we know that if somebody with brown eyes partners with somebody with blue eyes, they're very likely to have a brown-eyed child because the genes for brown eyes are more commonly expressed. But there are many things that are very complex that we don't always understand as well, particularly many types of mental illness. The risk for mental illness is multifactorial, meaning it can happen when gene issues and environmental issues combine to affect the function of our most important organ— our brain. We do know that we can cut down the risk of mental illness and heritable medical issues by avoiding donors with those issues in their family, which is one reason we emphasize the proper psychological screening and genetic counseling and, if possible, choosing a donor who has extensive family history available and multiple siblings. The more information you have, the better decision you can make. Sometimes gaining information can complicate a decision you previously felt good about, as in the following story, but in the end, you want to feel confident about your future child's health. What you want for your future child is for them to be healthy first.

WENDY AND BRAD

Wendy and Brad were considering an egg donor who seemed to check many of the boxes they wanted in a donor, not least of which was the fact that she had donated four times previously, and those dona-tions had been successful in leading to live births. She also played the flute in a local symphony, and finding a donor with artistic talent was an impor-tant factor for the couple. However, this donor had never spoken to a genetic counselor. And when she completed her genetic counseling interview at our clinic, it was discovered that she had a congenital (found at birth) malformation of her heart that needed to be corrected at age twelve. The interview also revealed other possible cardiac history within her family. None of this was in her written history, so it was new information. Congenital birth defects can be significant, and cardiac defects can affect children most dramatically.

Wendy and Brad held each other's hands in a tight grip as they talked with their genetic counselor about the risks. They still felt a strong connection with this donor, and the idea of starting over with their search felt deflating. They sought counseling to weigh the pros and cons and discuss their feel-ings. Ultimately, they decided not to work with her because they were told there was a 7–10 percent risk of passing on a life-altering cardiac defect to their child. As Wendy said, "It's both a really hard and really easy decision."

At Illume Fertility, every egg donor we interview not only reports their history but also spends forty-five minutes to an hour talking to a genetic counselor who will complete a family tree and look into their family history. In doing this, the counselor's eye is focused on the cause of death of all their relatives, any history of cancer and other medical illnesses, and also their general well-being and characteristics, such as height and weight. Genetic counselors are also trained to consider polygenic and multifactorial issues that relate to adult diseases, such as diabetes, high blood pressure, or bowel diseases. You can see why it's so important that family history is corroborated by a genetic counselor. That's why we do not recommend working with an egg or sperm donor who was adopted, because we don't have this history at all. We would be missing half the information about the health issue that could play into the future health of your child.

And that is our advice to you, whether you are seeking an egg donor or a sperm donor. Be clear with your clinic that a genetic counseling session has been completed so that you and the clinic understand the family tree. As an aside, it's a great idea to keep this family tree so it's available for your child-to-be. At some point, you'll be talking with your child about their donor's medical information, and it would be nice to have as much information as possible on the family tree of their donor. A premade family tree is available in *My Lifebook,* which will be discussed later in the book.

Cross-Check with the Patient's Genetics

While genetic counselors talk about things that are mostly polygenic, such as cancers, mental illness, or heart disease, we do have some very detailed tests now that look for single-gene errors, such as sickle cell disease, Tay-Sachs, or cystic fibrosis. And it's important to conduct these panels on both the donor and the parent who will be genetically linked to the child.

When we started working in reproductive medicine more than thirty years ago, we did no genetic testing on couples with infertility. We just tried to help them get pregnant. Then it was discovered that cystic fibrosis was present in one out of every thirty people of Caucasian ancestry, and so we began to offer panels looking for people who were carriers for cystic fibrosis and other common gene errors. Early on, we offered seven recessive gene panels (gene mutations that are known to cause disease if the child inherited one of the mutations from each parent), then we went to fifty-gene panels, to sixty-five, to seventy-five, and so on. Now the panel of recessive gene screening is up to five hundred to six hundred genes. This is important because 70–80 percent of us have genes for a disease in our genetic closet—anything from cystic fibrosis to things you probably haven't heard of, like mucolipidosis type 4.

But thankfully, human beings get their genes from two sources, sperm and egg, and the gene for most of these inheritable diseases must be present on both sides to express that disease. That's why we check both the donor and the parent. If the person on one side of the equation is a carrier for a disease—something that might only be present in one out of five thousand people—then you want to make sure that the person on the other side is not. Otherwise, your child that you've worked so hard to have has a 25 percent chance of having that disease. Some of these genes that we screen for are not that severe and can possibly be modified by different diets or lifestyle choices, but most of them are life-changing conditions. You can see why having a panel for recessive genes that cause disease on both the egg source and the sperm source is truly essential for parents-to-be. In fact, we believe that in the future, even people who are planning to conceive naturally will proactively get a panel looking for genetic diseases in their genetic closet so they're aware of whether they need to pursue advanced testing to avoid a disease.

Previously, we said that if the parent has condition A and the donor has condition A, then the child is going to have a 25 percent risk of having that disease, but it actually gets more complicated than that. Some genetic disorders, such as hemoglobinopathies (disorders of the hemoglobin molecule, which carries oxygen in our red blood cells), can result when there is not the same mutation on both sides but two different mutations that, when put together, could lead to a severely affected child. Of course, you don't have to understand all these possible combinations! But this is why it's important to have a meeting with a genetic counselor after completing genetic testing on yourself and on your donor, just to triply confirm that you're making the best choice.

Certainly, it could make you very sad if you have to give up a donor you've become attached to due to a genetic risk, but we would never recommend taking that risk in your child-to-be when it could be avoided. It is always heart-wrenching for us, too, when we have a patient who has fallen in love with a donor but has to make a different decision for genetic reasons, but the potential for heartbreak in the future is too great to risk it.

There may be times when you don't necessarily have to rule out a donor based on a matching genetic risk. In situations where we're fortunate to have a familial match—where a sister is donating to a gay brother's partner, or a sister is donating to a sister—and where we have full access to the sibling's family tree, we may go forward with the donation even if there is a match in a disease-causing gene. In that case, we can use advanced embryo-screening technology to find out whether both of the broken genes are present in the embryo or not. And we would only choose to transfer an embryo that has neither of the two broken genes or just one, but never two, because if we transfer an embryo with two recessive genes, the child would have a nearly 100 percent chance of having that disease process. The technology is called *preimplantation genetic testing for monogenic diseases* (PGT-M).

Consider the Personal Health History of the Donor

After family history and genetics, you will want to look closely at the personal health history of the gamete donor. Are they of a healthy weight? Do they have, perhaps, ADHD or difficulty in maintaining school achievement? Do they, or did they, have high cholesterol? We will discuss more of this later when we help you organize your priorities in choosing a donor and rank issues in order of importance.

Much of this information is going to be included in their profile, but remember that their profile is self-reported, and that's why it's important that any egg source or sperm source also be screened by a medical professional. (It's also important to use proper psychological screening, which we'll talk more about in chapter 7, not only to screen for psychopathology but also to get a sense about this person and whether they are likely to be truthful.) Medical clearance of egg or sperm donors includes a physical exam and an assessment of their overall health. Egg donors historically have been more scrutinized than sperm donors because the level of medical intervention necessary for them to donate their eggs is greater, since they're given medication and go through a procedure to have their eggs retrieved. But sperm donors should be screened just as carefully.

A donor's body weight can provide important insight. If a donor reports a very low BMI, it may be a sign that they have an eating disorder. Even if they don't, someone who is underweight may not make great sperm or eggs. It's important to look at this in the context of their family history. Let's say everyone in their family is extra lean. In that case, it's often just genetics and not necessarily something to worry about. But if they're an outlier in their family, it might be an indicator of their well-being. The same is true of donors who are beyond their optimal weight. Our observation is that you should try to work with a donor who is a normal weight—someone who lands within the range of 20–25 BMI.

You may also look at whether the donor reports needing tubes in their ears as a child, multiple dental surgeries, or having had a hernia. Donors are usually people under thirty, so needing surgeries to address issues at that young age may be an indicator of risk. You may not want to exclude a donor based on their need for small surgeries, but it is certainly something to put into the rubric.

Find Out About Lifestyle Choices

It's also important to consider your donor's health choices—how they choose to live their lives. When we evaluate donors, we are looking for the difficulties that they can pass on to a future child, and we're also looking at their ability to endure treatment and produce a large number of healthy eggs. A top consideration for both of these is whether the donor has a history of using substances that are not friendly to fertility.

While discussing how the patient should prepare for

pregnancy in the previous chapter, we mentioned research that looks at substance use and its effect on pregnancy success rates. The information gleaned there applies to donors as well. The data shows that any amount of smoking is associated with lower success. We all know that smoking is bad for you, and it's logical that it would be associated with poorer reproductive outcomes. We have much less information on smoking cannabis but we do know that when you inhale any superheated gas, your body has to choose to defend itself from reactive oxygen species, or breakdowns of that superheated gas. Because sperm and egg cells are in division and making new combinations of DNA, we have concerns about inhaling any superheated gas for its potential to break DNA and affect the potential success of an embryo-to-be. That likely includes vaping. We don't have any information on the effects of edibles, but we will reject donors who have any evidence of THC in their system because we don't want them smoking anything, and we don't know if we can wholly trust that someone is only ingesting cannabis and not smoking it. There is not a lot of information on the effect of THC itself on reproductive outcomes, but the safest decision is to avoid it before and during pregnancy.

Past substance use does not have to automatically rule out a donor, however. The eggs in an egg donor's ovary are protected from the bloodstream up until the months prior to the development of the eggs for ovulation. We consider this development cycle to be approximately three months, and environmental exposures come more into play the closer we get to the active follicular development cycle. This means if we encounter a donor who otherwise looks good but might have lifestyle choices like alcohol and tobacco use that we think are not helpful, we can ask them to stop their use completely or reduce it dramatically for three months prior to donation.

Similarly, the sperm development cycle is about seventy to ninety days, during which time it develops from a very immature sperm into a fully mature sperm with a compacted head. The mature head contains the genetic code for twenty-three chromosomes and energy cells to power its tail so that it can swim through the reproductive tract. Considering the sperm development cycle of approximately three months, men can reset their sperm quality in that amount of time through lifestyle choices. So once again, if you're using a known sperm donor—a family member or perhaps a designated sperm donor—we think it's important to ask that person to be eating well, not smoking at all, and not drinking frequently for those three months before donation. They also should not be using performance-enhancing drugs.

And what about eating well? The tips in the previous chapter about preparing for pregnancy apply here as well. As you probably know, our food stream in our modern world is very complex and is not what humans were meant to eat. All the sugars and fat, as well as the herbicides and pesticides and other chemicals in our food stream, likely can affect our gametes, so it's important to consider how your donor eats. I (Mark) do ask every donor I see what they eat, and I don't like to hear they mostly eat fast food and takeout. It can be difficult to draw a hard line on the eating choices for your donor, partly because it's tough to say exactly where that line should be, but we just want to make sure it's not well outside the norm.

Factor in the Donor's History of Donating

We alluded to this earlier in the chapter: A particular donor's history of success is also a consideration. For example, even though sperm is probably only 10–20 percent of the equation for success, using a sperm source that has never been used by anybody else before requires a leap of faith, simply because we don't know how successful that person's sperm can be. Alternatively, if you can find a sperm donor who has generated several pregnancies or children before, that can be very reassuring, and that sperm source has a leg up on someone who has never had a pregnancy success. That doesn't mean that you should automatically reject a sperm source that has never been used before or never successfully been used before. If all the other testing and genetics are normal, you can feel comfortable moving forward with that sperm source. Previous success is only one factor.

You may choose to weigh the importance of previous success a bit less if you're using an egg donor as opposed to a sperm donor, simply because the number of times a woman can donate is limited. Donating eggs is a much more significant commitment than providing a sperm donation.

Egg donors not only have more rigorous screening because of their medical commitment, their time commitment to donate their eggs is also upward of three weeks. And during those three weeks, your donor will be taking fertility medicines, becoming bloated and uncomfortable, and facing a risk of bleeding and infection and damage to her own fertility. This is one of the reasons the American Society for Reproductive Medicine guidelines recommend limiting women to a maximum of six donations. If you're looking at a fresh donor, and she's never donated before, and all her markers look good, then you can certainly move forward with her. On the other hand, if you can find an egg source who has donated before and has generated a good amount of eggs retrieved (perhaps fifteen or more), and you can access the information on embryo quality and outcome of pregnancy, then that donor might be more desirable than one who has never donated before.

At the end of the day, finding an experienced donor, whether it's a sperm donor or an egg donor, with proven outcomes is an advantage. In our opinion, if you're choosing between two donors, one you might like better in terms of looks or grade point average or eye color, and one who has proven outcomes, remember that you're trying to have a baby, and all things being equal, you may want to consider the one with the proven outcomes. Those traits and features that you've attached some emotional importance to may not even come to fruition in your child in the complex interplay of genes and environment, but a record of successful live births is a more reliable marker for your success.

A Discussion About Sperm Banks

You read about vitrification, or the cryopreservation of human eggs, in chapter 2. The effort to cryopreserve human eggs to help women preserve their fertility had been a holy grail for many years, since the introduction of assistive reproductive technologies. The efforts toward preserving eggs using the same method we use to cryopreserve other cells unfortunately were not successful in generating viable embryos that made pregnancies beyond a rate of 20–30 percent. But vitrification changed that. By introducing sugar molecules into the fluid surrounding the egg before the freezing process, we help protect the egg and keep it viable when it is plunged into liquid nitrogen and brought to a temperature of −197 degrees Celsius. This means that we now have the ability to freeze a human egg, and upward of 60–80 percent of the time, that egg survives the cryopreservation process and can move on and have the opportunity to be fertilized and hopefully create a healthy embryo.

Like an egg, a sperm is a single cell. But unlike an egg, which is mostly water, a sperm is the smallest cell in the human body, and most of the water has been pushed out of it. That makes sperm much more resilient as it goes through the cryopreservation process. So, whereas using frozen eggs results in a lower live birth rate compared to using fresh donor eggs, the data shows that using previously frozen sperm does not have a lower success rate compared to sperm that hasn't been frozen. We do lose a percentage of sperm in the freeze/thaw process, but because a single vial of frozen sperm typically has five million to ten million sperm in it, that loss is essentially meaningless. Even if we lose 50 percent in the vial, we still have enough sperm to generate a conception and hopefully a healthy pregnancy and child.

And that means you can feel very confident about using previously frozen sperm, though there *are* situations where that is not optimal. For example, if someone is choosing to use a known donor such as a family member as a sperm source and that donor has an abnormal (low) sperm count, the sperm cryopreservation process may result in too great an attrition rate. In that case, a fresh sperm specimen will likely be recommended. Thankfully, this is a relatively rare situation, and those particular persons donating sperm would never be chosen as a sperm donor at a sperm bank. Any donor to a sperm bank will have a sperm count in the normal range.

MARIO III

Mario III was a young man who came to see us with a diagnosis of azoospermia, or nonviable sperm. He was one of two boys from a very traditional Italian family. He and his brother were both married, and his brother had children while Mario and his wife, Cathy, did not. They had been trying for years with no success, and by the time they came to the clinic, they had visited several doctors, tried medication and surgery, and were emotionally and financially spent.

Mario III was a kind young man who felt very proud of his heritage and close to his family. He wrote his *III* on all his paperwork and explained how difficult his grandparents' immigration was and how they had built their family business (where he and his brother worked) from "nothing." The whole extended family always got together for holidays and Sunday night dinners, and the older folks were excited to bring a new generation of children into the fold.

For Mario III, the idea of using sperm from an unknown source felt devastating, so he asked his brother, Joe, who agreed. However, Cathy was nearing ovarian decline, and the time-consuming testing and process to screen his brother made her anxious and created an enormous amount of stress for the couple. There were times when she had trouble going to work. She wanted her husband, whom she adored, to be able to use family genetics, but every moment felt like a race against the clock. To make matters worse, Joe did not have a perfect sperm count either, though it was much better than Mario III's.

Mario III and Cathy engaged in individual and couple's counseling, and that helped them manage the multiple appointments, the wait, and the un-known. Still, they worried: What if after all of this it didn't work? What if it all took too long and Cathy's eggs were too old? These fears often felt consuming. Fortunately, after some treatment and a few attempts, Joe was able to produce a sperm sample that eventually helped to create a few healthy embryos. Cathy is now pregnant with their second child. The entire family is overjoyed.

Many families would not go to these lengths to produce sperm (or eggs) that may not create a healthy embryo, especially if the person with the ovaries felt her fertility potential was narrowing. For Mario III and Cathy, it was worth it. They understood the risk, they had extensive counseling, and their family supported any choice they made. Mario III's parents even suggested adoption at one point because it was so difficult to watch their son and daughter-in-law struggle. Yet the ultimate decision came down to Mario III and Cathy. Fortunately, it all worked out well.

Sperm banks are a tremendous resource for couples needing that gamete to help them complete the process, but you need to be diligent in choosing your sperm bank and your sperm donor because not all sperm banks fully screen donors for mental health, recessive genes, and medical issues.

Historically, sperm donors were never as fully screened as egg donors, and we are still catching up in that regard.

The bottom line is that there are many sperm banks out there to choose from, but not all are doing comprehensive screening on sperm donors, so our message is: Parents-to-be, beware. You're giving your child the genetics of that sperm source. Be just as thoughtful about it as someone choosing an egg donor.

Be Diligent (And Use the Help Available to You)

It may sound obvious, but it's important to recognize that your donor's family history and some of their traits will be passed on to your child. That's why these medical considerations are so critical, and why both sperm donors and egg donors should be screened thoroughly. Be diligent in looking at these factors—they are not details that can be let go. In addition, we strongly advise you to get the help of appropriate genetic counseling, mental health counseling, and medical counseling when looking at potential donors. These professionals are invaluable in helping you decide whether a particular donor is the best choice for you.

5

Anonymous, Open, and Known Donors

Patients tend to have many questions and varying comfort levels around donor openness. Unfortunately, there is also a wide range of conflicting opinions on the subject. But those of us who have remained abreast of the research and have seen thousands of recipients and donors over the decades know that the main thing people need is a solid, basic education on the topic so they can make an informed decision and avoid regret. We see every day how grateful, relieved, and satisfied people are when they have the information they need.

This subject is sensitive for many people, and it is also evolving, so we urge you to factor the information in this chapter into your decision-making process but also stay on top of the research. At the time of this writing, these terms have already changed. However, these are the terms that are most commonly used and understood, so for the sake of clarity, we will use the outdated terms *anonymous, open,* and *known.* We suspect that many more changes in this arena will emerge over the next decade.

Open Versus Anonymous Donors

More and more, people are interested in having the option to connect with their donor at some point in the future and are taking advantage of this option. However, because this trend has become more common only in the last few years, the majority of donations to date have been anonymous. We are often asked if it is important to choose an open donor. The answer is that it would be ideal, but it is complicated for several reasons, which we will get into as we look at all the options that may be available to you.

The least open option is an anonymous donor who indicated at the time of donation that they do not want to be contacted at any point. In practical terms, of course, anonymity is impossible in today's world. With the availability of resources such as 23andMe and Ancestry.com, people are finding genetic relatives more easily than ever. Facebook and other platforms offer facial recognition, and Google tells us what we want for breakfast! Well, that last one isn't true, but by the time your child grows up, many more advances such as retinal recognition may be available. At the time of this writing, one US state just passed legislation that gives recipients access to their donor information.

Yes, it is truly not possible to be anonymous anymore: Anyone who is genetically linked to another family tree may be able to find those people and contact them. If your donor did not agree to be contacted, there still may be a small chance that your child will receive a warm welcome if they contact that person many years later. Some donors do change their minds, but you obviously can't count on that.

There are varying degrees of open options in egg and sperm donation. Many egg donor agencies, and some clinics, provide options for openness or a range of semi-open options. These options might include the donor being willing to be reached out to for medical information, providing ongoing information to the attorney to share with you, having a relationship with you in the present or future, or having a relationship with your child in the present or future. Sperm banks and egg banks do not provide full openness (when the donor and intended parents exchange personal contact information and agree to communicate directly with each other) but often provide an option to reach out to the donor or obtain information about them when the donor-conceived child turns eighteen.

If your donor agreed to talk to your child when your child turns eighteen, we suspect they will honor that agreement. However, when these donors donate their gametes, they are often young and (even with some counseling) may not be thinking about (or counseled enough about) how it will feel to speak to (possibly) hundreds of offspring decades later. If your child is the tenth child to reach out to your sperm donor, the donor may be more likely to answer their questions than if your child is the hundredth person reaching out to that donor. This is something you will need to prepare your child for if they are interested in meeting their donor.

This raises the question: Will your child be interested in meeting their donor? Many are, and it's ideal to give them that option, but of course you can't predict the future, as you can see in the following patient stories.

REENA AND STEVE

Reena and Steve wanted to have two children, but Steve had suffered an injury in the marines that left him impotent. After considering all their options, they adopted one boy and had a second son with donor sperm. Both of those children are now in their twenties. The adopted son wanted to know more about his birth mom and pursued that information, even arranging to meet her. Since then, he and his birth mom have stayed in touch by email. In contrast, the son who was born through donor sperm has shown no interest in knowing more about the man who donated his sperm to his parents so he could come into existence, even though Reena and Steve were honest about his history from an early age and did everything they could to keep every door open. If this young man changes his mind in the future, he will have that option because his parents chose an open donor.

———

KATE AND CHLOE

Kate and Chloe were twin girls who were very close. They joined the same clubs in school, shared some of the same friends, and had a strong bond. Until recently, they also felt similarly about their donor. Their parents had spoken to them about their donor from the time they were very young, and it was "not a big deal" for either of the girls. They were very comfortable with the idea, and although the subject came up periodically, they mostly focused on their day-to-day lives.

When it was time for college, they began talking more about their donor. We often see children explore their histories more when they move away from home, so this was not unusual. What was surprising was that now Kate wanted to meet her do-nor, while Chloe was not interested. Their parents sent them to me (Lisa) to talk through their feelings.

As we got to know one another in my office, Chloe made a couple of jokes early on to help her and her sister feel more comfortable talking about this important subject. Kate was friendly, but she wanted to get down to brass tacks: "I want to meet our donor to see if we have similar interests—maybe she studied humanities in college like I'm going to," she said. She poked a finger into a hole in her jeans. "And, I don't know, I want to see if we look alike, or if she went on to have children of her own." Chloe said she was not opposed to meeting, nor did she feel particularly driven or curious. She felt that the information her parents had shared with her and the information she and Kate had received from 23andMe was sufficient. She said she would sup-port Kate in her search, but she didn't think she would join her in a potential meeting.

In the end, Kate decided to delay the meeting. Though she had the support of her sister and par-ents, she had hoped that she and Chloe would find and meet their donor together. For now, she will wait for a while and see if Chloe develops more in-terest over time. If she doesn't, Kate is prepared to search on her own.

Your child may or may not be interested in meeting their donor, and your donor may or may not be enthusiastic about meeting your child. Choosing an open donor gives you the opportunity to tell your child that they have the option, and then you can help prepare them for the possibilities that lie ahead. Your child may have fantasies about what that donor is like, and those fantasies may or may not match the reality. If your child is interested in searching, it's helpful to work with a specialist who can help you support your child and prepare them for what they may find on the other side of their questions. Some people will feel a connection with their donor, some will feel disappointment, and others will feel relief. Most will have a mix of feelings. What's most important is to be your child's ally in their self-discovery—to help them navigate the bumps in the road and hold their hand while they explore their connections.

The uncertainty of not knowing how a donor will react to requests for contact in the future can feel stressful for many parents-to-be who want to provide their future child with every option available. However, you must feel good about the donor with regard to their medical and family history as described in the previous chapter—it may not be possible to find a donor who is the right match for your family and is also willing to be open. One day, it's likely that all gamete donations will be open. Until then, you will need to accept the limitations of the world we live in and make the best choice you can with the information you have available.

Open Versus Known Donors

The words *open* and *known* are often used interchangeably, but in this book, we use the term *open donor* to refer to a donor who is anonymous to you but is willing to be open in some way or at some point in time. A *known donor* is someone who is known to you prior to the donation process, like a friend or family member.

Though an open donor is not initially known to the recipients, they may agree to future contact and may develop a relationship with your family over time. This person would have been recruited by an agency or a clinic to donate their eggs. In the case of sperm donation, the men who donate their sperm have the option to indicate their willingness to meet the offspring when the offspring are eighteen. Sperm banks have a large number of donors, so arranging specific plans with your donor through the bank will probably not be an option. This may change over time as more people become interested in some level of openness with their donor, but right now it's not possible to have a fully open relationship with your sperm donor if you use a sperm bank.

An egg donor recruited from a clinic or agency may be willing to stay in touch, send and/or receive pictures, or communicate when medical information is needed. You and your donor will agree on these plans early in the process. When you do, you will likely exchange contact information or agree to communicate through your agency or attorney, and agree upon the level of contact you will have and when it can happen. You may choose to arrange contact directly or through your attorney. Everyone's comfort level is different, and therefore the level of openness that each family desires may be different. So while it's always of primary importance to think about what the child may want in the future and how you can consider their best interests, you must also find a donor with whom you feel comfortable and who can provide you with the best chance of having a healthy child.

Once you and your donor have come to an agreement, you should discuss it with your attorney and have them draw up your contract. Some patients create simple contracts, and others design elaborate agreements that include video libraries for the future child. I (Lisa) have helped many patients plan a wide range of mutually beneficial arrangements with their donors and have had wonderful experiences as a result.

EAST VERSUS WEST

There is a great divide between the East and West Coast in the United States with regard to gamete donation. Donors on the West Coast are frequently open or known, whereas East Coast donors have historically been anonymous. At Illume Fertility and Gay Parents to Be, we created an open donor program. It is an unusual program on the East Coast, and we are grateful to the partners and CEO, Robin

Mangieri, who had the courage and insight to support this idea.

Unlike an open donor, a known donor is typically a friend or a family member who offers to donate eggs or sperm to the individual or couple that is trying to build a family, like Mario III's brother (page 118). These arrangements are becoming increasingly common, and although they can be an ideal situation for many people, they can also be problematic. Often, parents-to-be go into the arrangement with the best of intentions and later discover problems they did not foresee. One concern is that the goals of everyone in the relationship may not be in alignment. Another is that, as close as you may be now, mutual respect or interest may evaporate over the years.

Think of it this way: People go into marriages with the best of intentions and plans for the future, and yet many couples divorce. These people are in love, they often share similar values and perspectives on child-rearing and the world, and they share an intimate relationship that helps fuel their desire to work things out when they have disagreements. Yet even with that bedrock of commitment under them, they still may reach a point where they decide the best solution is divorce. Now imagine how difficult it may be to negotiate with someone in a less committed, less robust relationship, like a friend or relative you are co-parenting with. You may have a complicated history with this person, or their plans for the future may diverge from yours, or their views may conflict with yours—even if they seem totally aligned now. Either of you may want to move away or begin new relationships. So much can happen over time. We have seen many co-parenting or known donor situations work out beautifully, but not without a good deal of work in counseling, where they can hammer out details that may have never occurred to them.

For these reasons and more, it's essential to speak with an experienced therapist who has been well trained to help you map out the potential pros and cons in advance and determine if the relationship will be manageable. Together, you may identify areas for concern but feel able to navigate them, or you may discover there are just too many concerns to pursue using a friend or family member as a donor. Through this process, it is vitally important to remember each decision needs to consider the best interests of the child.

At the Center for Family Building, and at Illume Fertility, I (Lisa) meet with the donor and their partner (if applicable) to perform psychological screening, conduct a psychological interview, and assess their readiness to donate. Then we help them think about possible issues that may arise in the future. Based on their history, the recipient's history, their relationship with each other and their family and friends, and many other factors, we discuss their views on many scenarios that may cause concern down the road. Then I meet with the recipient and their partner, review their histories, and cover similar topics. Finally, I meet with all parties together to review any potential conflicts, concerns, or insights that have become evident in the course of the counseling sessions so all parties can leave the meeting with specific plans for the future and a clear sense of topics to include in their legal contract. These topics are important to hammer out early because they will inform many issues that will be relevant in their future.

Plan for the Unforeseen with a Contract

Speaking of contracts, what should be in yours? That's something you will want to work out with your attorney after detailed conversations with your therapist, but in general, agreements can include information about a wide range of things. Many open donor contracts include a request for the donor to reach out with updated medical information. Many donors are young and healthy when they donate, but health changes over time. Would you like to receive medical updates directly? And what if the clinic or your attorney is not in business in twenty years? Do you have another way to connect with each other? Perhaps you would like to set up a specific email address where you can reach each other for any purpose you agree upon. Maybe you both want to agree to sign up with the Donor Sibling Registry (a wonderful registry for donor-conceived siblings, which we will get into later), or maybe you want to share personal contact information. Everyone's idea of what feels good for their family is different. What's important is to think through these things early in the game if possible. A little hard work spent on this at the beginning can save you frustration, disappointment, and more down the road.

Contracts with a donor you know often address many topics, such as who will spend time with the child, an agreement on the disposition of unused embryos, financial obligations for the future child, and plans for a guardian in the event that something happens to one or both parents. People also include specific plans such as how many times the donor will donate and how many children can be created as a result of the donation. Issues laid out in co-parenting agreements can be similar to issues seen in divorce agreements, such as how you will manage your relationship with the child if one of you leaves the country, who will take the children for holidays, and how you will handle issues such as religion, finances, and education. It will be important to consider how you negotiate and the dynamics in your relationship, because negotiation will be a skill that you will be using a great deal over the years.

These contracts can be very detailed or very vague. In our experience, the more detailed contracts are preferable. Although some facets of these contracts may not be enforceable or guaranteed to hold up in court, they can be very useful and give you some measure of security as well as a framework for everyone to live by.

We believe it is essential to ensure that the series of meetings we described is conducted. Sometimes patients tell us they don't need these meetings—they feel they can figure it out on their own, or they have such a close relationship that they don't need to worry—but this subject, like many in this book, reminds us of the old saying that a fish doesn't know it's in water. In other words, being in the midst of this exciting moment can make it difficult to be aware of its potential pitfalls. Does this mean it's always complicated and difficult to come to an agreement? No. These agreements often work out well, and many different family arrangements can be thoughtful and loving. But you do need to sort through ideas that you may not have thought of and consider issues you may be missing. Doing so gives you the best chance of building a good and unified family for your future child.

Consider the following story about an agreement that went south.

JENNIFER, HEATHER, AND JEREMY

When Jennifer and Heather decided they wanted to have children, they considered themselves lucky to have a mutual friend, Jeremy, who was willing to donate his sperm. He was healthy, smart, and good-looking, and his family history didn't show any genetic concerns, so it seemed like a great match. Jeremy wanted to help them, and he was not interested in co-parenting or being a part of the lives of the children, which worked for Jennifer and Heather. They knew that when the children were older, they could reach out to him if they desired.

After donation, Heather went on to have twins,

and as agreed, Jeremy did not have a relationship with these children. However, he did send them a birthday card each year, which he signed, "Love, Dad." He simply wanted the children to know that he was thinking of them. When the children went to college, the moms asked Jeremy to help pay for tuition. Because he had not co-parented or been a part of the family in any way, he refused. When he did, Jennifer and Heather sued him for tuition money— and won. To the court, just writing "Dad" on the card meant that he was claiming parentage.

This is just one example of a situation that nobody would have predicted at the beginning, and it had a painful effect on this family. We have seen other situations where family members stop speaking to one another, where people go to court over custody of embryos, and where religious or cultural preferences make the process of treatment and parenting arrangements problematic. Remember that it is vitally important to consider the effects these decisions will have on your future child or children. An experienced counselor can help you avoid some of the problems that others have had before you.

As we have said, though, a carefully planned agreement can work out quite well, as the following story shows.

JEANNETTE AND IVAN

Jeannette was a single heterosexual teacher who always wanted to marry and have children but never did. Her friend Ivan was a married gay man who wanted children but whose husband kept delaying because of the difficulty and cost of the surrogacy process. Sadly, shortly after Ivan's husband agreed to start the process of donor conception, he developed an aggressive form of cancer and passed away. Ivan was devastated and never remarried—but he did continue to long for a child.

One evening, Ivan and Jeannette got to chatting at a party, and Jeannette happened to mention how much she longed to be a mother. "Oh my goodness. Me, too!" Ivan replied excitedly, causing a few heads to turn their way. The two ignored the attention and kept talking. Jeannette was self-supporting but not wealthy and had a very demanding schedule. Ivan, on the other hand, had done well financially and was semiretired. As they talked, a plan began to form. They had several meetings with me (Lisa) and talked it through some more, and they kept talking about it over the next few weeks. Eventually, they both agreed they would be a great match.

In our sessions, we discussed what they each wanted their day-to-day lives to look like, how they

> would spend holidays, and how they would make decisions about finances, schooling, activities, and more. We talked about their plans for disclosure to the child and their friends and families, and we talked about how they would manage these issues if either married, had other children, or moved away. Among the many issues we discussed were topics such as paying for treatment, how long treatment would continue, how many children they would have, and plans for the pregnancy and delivery. These friends put in a lot of time to work out a lot of details, and that time was well spent.

An old quote has been attributed to an anonymous woodsman who was asked, "What would you do if you had just five minutes to chop down a tree?" He answered, "I would spend the first two and a half minutes sharpening my axe." We can't foresee where life will take us, but preparing rigorously gives us the best chance to successfully handle problems that arise.

Fortunately, we have learned a lot since the development of modern sperm banks and since the first donor-egg baby was born in 1983. As the number of donor-conceived children grows, we will continue to expand our understanding of donor conception and the effects that these scientific miracles have had on the lives of the recipients, offspring, and donors. When that time comes, there will likely be more research and a more collective understanding of the best elements to include in a contract. We will be more informed about issues that frequently come up in court cases and decisions that should be made for the best interest of the child.

A Move Toward Openness

When we started in reproductive medicine, all donors were anonymous. Over the past thirty years in the donor-conception world, the pendulum has swung from 100 percent anonymous to increasing degrees of open and known, particularly among egg donors. There are very few open sperm donors out there compared to known egg donors. Some of that may relate to the ease of donating sperm compared to donating eggs, and some of that may relate to the motivation of young men who choose to donate sperm compared to young women who choose to donate eggs. We've seen over a thousand egg donors over the years, and while some of them are surely on this journey at least partly because of their financial compensation package, almost all of them are clearly sincere in their desire to help somebody else have a family. Still, the shift toward openness is happening for donations of both gametes.

For me (Mark), this shift isn't only a professional matter. Living in this modern world—where the opportunity to meet your donor and to have a legal agreement for future contact for your child is common—makes me somewhat sad the opportunity to meet our donor wasn't available to my husband and me when we chose our donor. We were fortunate to work with a donor, therapist, and attorney who allowed us to put in place a future-contact agreement for our children when they are eighteen. I wonder about the donor for my children—what she is doing now, if she has children, how many other times she has donated, if my children have half siblings. And I'm just the parent. I can only imagine that my children, who hold her genetics, will be even more curious at some point soon. I wish I could do more to help them answer those questions. I certainly understand that it might be scary for some to move forward with an open or known donor, but I also believe that part of our job as parents is to do the hard things. For people using donor gametes, one of the hard things may be to face the fear and humility of needing to use a donor.

Another hard thing may be choosing an open donor even if that complicates your search. Plenty of donors are willing to be open, and while it may be disappointing to rule out an otherwise great donor because they're not willing, the value of using an open donor—as long as she is healthy and fits with your unique family circumstances—is perhaps beyond quantifiable if your child really wants to know more.

As a therapist and mother of three nongenetically linked children, I (Lisa) admit I, like Mark, have a bias toward openness. I am keenly aware that children conceived with the assistance of egg or sperm donation will have different experiences from adopted children; I've observed this in my more than two decades of practice. I have also seen many similarities. But one of the key differences—and this is very important to remember—is that, at the time of the donation, the donors we have seen are not donating to parent your child. Children in the foster care system are often removed from families who wanted to parent but were unable to, and typically birth families who place their children at birth grieve over the loss of their child even when they understand they are making a good decision. Parents-to-be who are using a donor are often fearful that the donor will feel the same as a birth mother: They worry that the donor will feel like she is relinquishing a child and will have a strong desire to be active in the child's life. Ironically, donors often tell us they are also worried. They fear the parents will see them as a second mother. The donors we have seen are happy to help you grow your family but do not want to parent your child. They are not bonding with the eggs as they would a child they gave birth to. We commonly hear from donors something along the lines of: *I'm not using my eggs, and I'm not even sure if I want kids, so I may as well help someone else who really does want children but is unable to have them.* These donors often tell us that while they feel really good about helping an individual or couple build their families, they are also excited to continue with their careers, travel, or pursue whatever their personal goals are at the time they are donating. This does not mean that they may not be curious or interested in connecting with you at some point in the future if that is what you want, but they are very clear when they meet with us that their goal is to help someone else have a family, not become a parent themselves.

Yet many people are worried about establishing any level of openness. We often find ourselves reassuring both the donors and the intended parents that if they have an open relationship, their relationship will only reflect what they desire and what is laid out in their contract. The donor will not be obligated to more than they offer, and the intended parents will not be asked for more contact than they desire. Everyone may change over time and their relationship may develop, but at the time of donation, the contract will only reflect what all parties agree upon.

Another reason to consider an open donor is health and the reality that it changes over time. If your young, healthy donor develops breast cancer at age thirty-five, you may want that information so you can discuss early mammogram screenings with your daughter's doctor. It's true that advances in genetic testing are being made at lightning speed. Even so, it can be helpful to understand your child's genetics.

I (Lisa) once worked with a family whose daughter did not get her first tooth until she was two. Her pediatrician was perplexed and suggested some tests and perhaps a visit with a pediatric dentist who would take x-rays and determine the cause of these late-growing teeth. Before going through that, the parents contacted the donor, who told them that her teeth also came in late. While avoiding an x-ray does not seem major, it's one example of how even small issues could arise that could help a family understand their child's medical issue a bit more easily. And the fact is, not all clinics, agencies, or sperm or egg banks will continue to stay up to date with a donor's medical records. Most contracts ask the donors to reach out to their clinic or agency if they experience a health issue, but if you have an open relationship with your donor and you're able to find a way to stay in touch, you can more easily stay abreast of her health over time.

Here we need to emphasize the importance of using your medical and psychological team as you move forward. At the time of this writing, there have been multiple cases of donors selling their sperm online or attempting to donate sperm by having sex with the recipient. We don't need to tell you how potentially problematic this can be. It's hugely important to stay safe with strangers, ensure your donor is not a carrier for a disease or genetic ailment, and take the steps necessary to protect yourself legally.

Eye on the Future

One more thing to consider as you make your decision with your eye on the future. If we fast-forward to when your child is older and perhaps wants to connect with their donor, it's very possible that their donor will have many donor-conceived offspring who are reaching out to them. If you already have a connection to her, it may be easier to reconnect with her than if you are some stranger who comes out of the blue in twenty years. Right now, you may feel overwhelmed with treatment and think that you can help your child with that connection when the time comes. And that is true, and it may work out just fine. However, if you can go the extra mile now and arrange a scenario where you can have some contact with your donor here in the beginning, it's more likely that she will remember you when you set out to find her later. Even if the two of you agree on specific terms for your relationship, just creating that connection can leave the door open to other possibilities in the future. And you never know, you may both find your connection to be very worthwhile, even at the beginning.

An open relationship can also be beneficial for the donors. Donors often tell us that although they know they are helping a couple or individual have a child, they typically only experience the medical process. But when they see the faces of the lives they are changing, it adds another dimension for them and gives more meaning to their donation. If you're not able to do this, or if you're using a sperm donor, another possibility is to connect with the Donor Sibling Registry so you can be connected to donor-related siblings. Those people may be able to provide medical information and give your child a chance to see others who share their genetics.

Even with our decades of meeting with donors and recipients, we can't predict what your relationship with your donor will be like years from now. We can only work with the information we have, and that's why it's so important to walk through these decisions with a well-trained mental health professional who can help you understand possibilities that may not otherwise have occurred to you.

6

Balancing Practical and Emotional Considerations

In addition to the medical decisions involved in choosing a donor and the decision about openness, emotion is also going to play a role. That's unavoidable. Balancing the practical factors with the emotional factors can be a challenge. There is so much to know and so much conflicting information out there on the internet. Friends and family members often want to offer their points of view, making the process even more stressful. It's no wonder choosing a donor is difficult for many people. You are choosing one-half of the genetics for your future child (or children)! That is a big deal.

As we have discussed, many people, when faced with this hard decision, are tempted to choose donors who make them feel comfortable in some way. Maybe the donor looks like someone in your family or has the same sense of humor or hobbies as you or your partner. Maybe they share your cultural background, or perhaps they are simply very attractive or smart. While it's certainly fine to factor any of these characteristics into your decision, it's important to prioritize other, more consequential factors. How can you balance these practical aspects with your emotional needs? Let's start by looking at those emotions.

Understand Your Emotions

People can find themselves needing donors for a variety of reasons, and each individual's situation comes with its own complex emotional implications. Chapter 1 addresses, in a general way, the emotions that patients typically experience as they come to terms with using a donor. Let's look more closely at what you may be feeling as it comes time to choose your donor.

LGBTQIA+ Couples

For people entering the donor-conception process as part of the LGBTQIA+ community, choosing a donor can be exciting but often difficult as well. These patients sometimes say they feel like there is another person intruding on their lives, or that they wish they could have a child with their own genetics. If you could create a child with both of your genetics, that would be ideal. (Medicine is rapidly progressing toward this future! We have seen animals bred with two parents of the same sex, but this science is not ready for prime time in humans, at least not yet.)[1]

For other people, choosing a donor is not especially stressful. If that's the case for you, that's great, but be aware that you may have blind spots. A little planning and thinking through the factors discussed in this chapter can go a long way toward helping you choose as wisely as possible.

Infertility Patients

If you have experienced infertility, your frustration in choosing a donor is likely to be accompanied by hurt. Grief over not having the family you dreamed of is part of the process of accepting a donor. You may have begun your journey with fantasies of a child who perhaps looked like you or your partner, carried your family genetics and heritage, and possibly had traits you could point to that reminded you of yourself. For years, you may have been thinking ahead about names, due dates, and baby showers. Many of those dreams and fantasies are shattered when you learn you cannot use your genetics to conceive. Thoughts such as *I hope my child has my family's beautiful dark hair or my partner's dimples* can vanish overnight, and all those thoughts and hopes need to be grieved.

And for men who need to use a sperm donor to conceive with their partner, it can mean the loss of their lineage. Historically, in our male-dominated society, to have children was an affirmation of one's masculinity. For some men, agreeing to use donor sperm is a tremendous ego blow that is hard to recover from.

The grief and loss can be overwhelming, and working with a qualified mental health professional to process your feelings can be invaluable. The next chapter's step-by-step guidelines for choosing a donor will also help you be methodical and deliberate about your choice of donor so you can plan for your future family in a way that isn't only influenced by your emotions.

Single Parents-to-Be

Single parents-to-be may experience the additional pain of not having a partner. Some individuals prefer to parent alone, but many always assumed that they would parent with someone. If you fall into the latter group, you may have come to a stage in your life where you're ready to parent, and parenting without a partner is better than not parenting at all. You may meet a partner later—single parents often do—but since there is no guarantee, you need to wrap your mind around a new definition of family. This is no small feat. Respect your feelings of loss and grief if beginning the journey alone was not your first choice.

Those with Medical Issues

Patients who have had medical difficulties that left them unable to use their own genetics to conceive may feel that using a donor is a double whammy. Not only have they experienced prolonged feelings of pain and sadness due to their medical issue, but fertility treatments, which can feel unfair and invasive, often trigger memories of previous treatments. It can also feel increasingly difficult to withstand disappointment—

like getting kicked in the leg where it's already bruised. On the other hand, some patients feel gratitude to be able to have a child at all. These reactions vary and are often complex. If you need a donor for medical reasons, you could have a wide range of reactions, and none are wrong.

The Donor Is Not a Blueprint

All these individual experiences need to be valued and understood during the process of choosing a donor—not only because it is vitally important to acknowledge your feelings but also because how you feel may affect your choice. It's crucial to educate yourself about the ideas outlined in this chapter so you can make a clear decision. After you have thought about these considerations, if you still believe having a donor with dark hair is the most important criterion (because, for instance, dark hair is a family trait that has been passed down for generations from your long line of Greek relatives), that's your prerogative—but first make sure you understand all the factors that go into your choice and their implications. To paraphrase a commercial from the days when we were younger, "an educated consumer is the best customer."

In other words, it's one thing to carefully consider all the issues presented in this book and then make a decision that takes into account your personal preferences, but it's another to choose a donor based on personal preference alone. You may feel sad that using donor gametes will cost your child a connection to your heritage, but choosing a donor who makes you feel better about that now without addressing other important factors can lead to problems down the road. The good news is that those problems are largely preventable.

To begin, let's think about donor conception in a slightly different way from how you may have imagined. It's natural to think about the donor's characteristics as being part of your child's looks, intelligence, or temperament. However, we all know people who look or behave very differently from their family members. Think about Prince Harry and Prince William, Bill Clinton and his half brother, Renée Zellweger and her brother, or Ashton Kutcher and his brother. In these famous examples, we can see clearly that people can differ quite a bit from their siblings in looks, temperament, drive, and possibly even intelligence—a situation far from uncommon. You can probably think of many examples from the families you have known in your life.

This difference between siblings plays out in our families. I (Mark) am one of four boys with the same parents, all of whom have taken different paths—from doctor to accountant to engineer to warehouse worker. And for me (Lisa), not only are my sisters and I very different in our personalities, but we look nothing alike. I am petite with a straight frame, blond hair, and green eyes. The middle sister has dark hair and hazel eyes and is very tall with a large frame, and my youngest sister had blue eyes and light brown/reddish hair and a very curvy body.

The point is that often we look at the donor's appearance, temperament, or talents to give us a sense of what our future child may be inheriting. But these are things over which we have very little control. We all need to remember you are not getting your donor but a random distribution of traits and genes from their previous generations. For example, I (Lisa) recently screened an egg donor with blond hair and light eyes, and who had similar hobbies as I did when I was younger. If I needed a donor and decided to choose her because she looked like me and had the same interests, the results could have been much different from what I'd anticipated. As it turns out, she has three brothers with red hair who were all math majors in college! This is one more example of how our family tree is so important. When it comes to assembling your future child's genetic makeup, it's helpful to remember that you will receive qualities from your donor's family background, not just from your donor and your own personal family tree. You will have a new unique combination of fifty-two thousand genes, and only twenty-six thousand will be expressed at any one time.

Even when both parents use their genetics, it's not possible to predict what the child's interests or temperament will be.

JULIE

Julie and her husband, Ronnie, planned to have one genetically related child and wanted a girl. Julie described herself as "girly" and a "bookworm," and she very much wanted a daughter who was similar. "I can't wait to take my daughter for manicures and have tea parties," she said. "I daydream about spending hours in bookstores together." Because they were only having one child, Julie was determined to have the girl of her dreams.

She used fertility treatment and a genetic screening tool to screen the embryos. (While it's common to use this tool to look for abnormalities, it also gives patients the advantage of learning the sex of the embryos.) Of course, she was concerned about the health of her future child, but she was also intensely focused on having a girl. In the end, she did have her girl—but her daughter did not fit the dreams Julie originally had. From a very early age, it was clear this child was not going to wear dresses or party shoes. She is interested in working on a farm and has never had a manicure. She loves being outdoors, frequently has Band-Aids on her fingers, and has no interest in reading for fun. Although she has both of her parents' genetics, her personality is nothing like either of theirs. While this possibility may be hard to digest, it is a real possibility—including for those choosing donors. You cannot design the temperament, personality, or essence of your child. It is a combination of genes, environment, and gene expression.

Even when we understand on a logical level that two parents can produce offspring who are wildly different not only from one another but also from the parents, it can still be hard to fully accept the idea that we can't control for the characteristics we most desire in a child-to-be. In our clinic, we have even seen patients who are physicians and genetic counselors who tell us they understand this reality. Yet when they choose their donor, all logic goes out the window. The grief, the desire to replace oneself, the desire to choose certain characteristics or a specific heritage or family trait—all these can create a powerful pull.

We are not suggesting you should not choose a donor you like. In fact, there are several reasons why finding someone you like can make sense. For one thing, liking your donor can help you feel more comfortable with your decision, and it's easier to say nice things about your donor to your child if you like that person. Second, even if you have an anonymous agreement, someone who seems like a kind person may be more likely to answer questions you may have in the future if you are able to connect with them one day. Finally, your child will know that there is a part of them that is connected to someone out there in the world, and if they hear you easily saying nice things about their donor, they will know that goodness is inside them as well. What we are saying is that liking your donor is only one factor to consider. The next chapter presents a step-by-step process to help you separate some of the things over which you have some control from the things over which you have very little control. There is no foolproof process to ensure you get all you desire for your future child, but you can stack the odds in your favor for the best outcome possible by using this framework.

7

Choosing Your Donor

A Five-Step Process

Looking through donor profiles can be confusing and exhausting. Follow these steps, and by the time you finish, your choices will be much clearer. But keep in mind that this is a guide, not a rule list. Choosing a donor is a very personal and emotional decision and usually takes a few months. If you are making this decision with a partner, you will need to both feel comfortable, or as comfortable as possible, about your decision. One or both of you may need to make compromises, and one or both of you may also have some disappointment if you can't agree on a decision. If you need help making this decision, speaking with a qualified mental health professional who specializes in this field can be useful.

Step 1: Psychological Screening

The American Society for Reproductive Medicine has established guidelines for screening donors. The guidelines outline a number of tasks that should be performed by a qualified therapist (someone trained through, and a member of, the Mental Health Professional Group for the American Society for Reproductive Medicine) before accepting a donor. Included in those guidelines is a psychological interview conducted by a licensed mental health professional trained in reproductive medicine and psychological testing. The two tests that are most commonly used are the Personality Assessment Inventory (PAI) and the Minnesota Multiphasic Personality Inventory (MMPI), which screen for psychopathology.

The psychological interview and the test are important for many reasons. Some psychological difficulties have a genetic component, meaning they can be passed on to the child, which means you'll obviously want to avoid them. It is also important to know that the donor, particularly an egg donor, is emotionally stable and secure enough to endure the invasive and sometimes emotional or painful process of donation.

The psychological test also screens for deception. If the donor is trying to hide aspects of herself that she does not want us to see or is attempting to portray herself in an exceptionally favorable light, then we assume she may not be answering the rest of the test honestly. Therefore, we can't have an accurate picture of her psychological health. We also may assume she is not being honest to the clinic about the information she shares about her medical history.

The mental health professional should also look for altruistic motives. While donors are typically compensated, we don't want them to be doing it only for the money. Therefore, a donor who doesn't also donate because they want to help an individual or couple have a child will typically not be allowed to donate. Likewise, someone who has a financial hardship or is on public assistance generally would not be considered as a good candidate for donation. We want you to know that your donor has a true desire to help someone build their family.

In addition to being interviewed and tested, donors are also educated about the implications of their donation. Egg donors in particular need to understand the short-term implications and risks associated with the medical procedures, including how to manage their emotions if they have a reaction to the medication, how they will feel when they first begin giving themselves shots, and what the retrieval process will be like. We even counsel them on how to manage feeling bloated (stretchy pants are key!).

Both egg and sperm donors must also consider how their donation may have ripple effects into their future. Offspring may reach out to them, and this may have an impact on their lives and the lives of their families. Not all prospective donors have thought through these issues and may, after counseling, decide that donation is not something they would like to pursue. In our practice, only 5–7 percent of donors who apply actually become candidates for donation.

There is no way to account for every possibility, but this screening will give the mental health professional a degree of comfort to approve the donor for a particular program. Most clinics, agencies, and banks will follow these guidelines, but not all, so be sure to ask. Some might provide personality profiles or lengthy descriptions of the donor, but these are not the same thing. Personality assessments like the PAI and the MMPI are designed to look for things like emotional difficulties, high-risk behaviors, and a penchant for not being truthful. Personality profiles and other assessments that are often provided to prospective patients will not provide you with the best chance of choosing a psychologically healthy donor.

These decisions aren't always easy, but having information at least allows you to make an informed one.

ANNIE AND HAHN

Annie and Hahn were married for three years but had known each other for more than ten. Their marriage did not work out, but after they divorced, they remained friends. In fact, they knew each other's families well and would stop by on Easter or Thanksgiving.

Years after their divorce, Annie decided she wanted to have a child, and she asked Hahn to be the father. He agreed. They came to the clinic and began the process of screenings and consultations to work through the short- and long-term implications of their plan. In counseling, they worked through many topics, such as how they would handle co-parenting with new partners, who would spend holidays with the child, and who would make major and minor decisions about everything from medical issues to after-school classes. Which one of them would bear the financial burden, or how would they each contribute? What would they do with excess embryos? How would their friends and family react? The list goes on, and they seemed to be able to work out solutions to most issues.

Then Hahn underwent psychological screening, which included a psychological interview and the PAI. It turned out that Hahn had many of the symptoms of bipolar disorder. When Hahn learned of this, he immediately saw himself in the symptoms. When we spoke with Annie, she, too, recognized the symptoms in her ex-husband. She had always described Hahn as "moody at times" and said he had a lot of energy; these mood swings had been a challenge for her and were part of the reason they divorced.

She was faced with a difficult choice. The two of them had worked through so many details, and everything seemed to be perfect—except for that diagnosis. Annie understood her future child could be affected with the same psychological difficulty. After thinking about it for a few days, she made the wrenching decision to go with a different donor, one without this difficulty. This was an opportunity for Hahn to better understand his "mood swings" and get help. They finally decided they would continue with their co-parenting plans and use a sperm donor from a sperm bank.

Most egg donors are properly screened, but it is still important to ask, especially if you are using an agency. Some agencies employ mental health professionals and some do not. If you would like to have a clear and objective view of your donor, then you can request your donor undergo screening with an independent mental health professional. Sperm banks began appropriately screening donors years after rigorous egg donor screening was in place by fertility clinics, and some still don't. Even those that conduct screening may have only started recently, so if you are choosing a sperm donor, be sure to ask the sperm bank when they began psychological testing with either of the tests listed above. If your sperm bank only began this protocol on February 1, 2017, for example, you may want to only consider donors who donated after that date. You may not be able to request independent screening for your sperm donor, but the sperm banks we have seen that do perform psychological screening do a very good job of employing mental health professionals who are seasoned in this area and have decades of experience.

Step 2: Replicated Risks

When you fall in love with someone, you usually haven't quizzed them about their genetic makeup ahead of time, and most heterosexual couples attempt to conceive at home without thinking about their genes. However, as we have discussed, if the two partners are carriers for a genetic condition, it is possible to pass that problem on to their future child. The same is true when using a donor. If the genetically linked parent-to-be and your donor are carriers for the same genetic condition, your child could be affected by that disease.

Chapter 4 discusses the medical screening that is necessary for any potential donor to undergo. Because it takes both a sperm and an egg to make an embryo, it should be no surprise that the partner(s) who will be genetically linked to the child should also go through that screening before treatment begins. If screening reveals that both the donor and the genetically linked parent-to-be are carriers for the same difficulty, the clinic will suggest you use a different donor.

Your fertility clinic's role in helping you choose your donor ends after your genetic consultation. But you can take your investigation further by looking at the donor's family tree to determine if the health problems in the genetically linked parent's family are similar to significant health problems in the donor's family. It is true that some people live past one hundred, but all people die of something or have some difficulty in their family, even if they die of "old age." It's rare to find someone who has no history of cancer or heart disease or diabetes in their family, for example. Donors are typically young and healthy, but you can look for these health issues in their family. If people in the genetically linked partner's family have died of colon cancer, for example, and your donor also has colon cancer in their family, you may be increasing the risk for your child.

We should point out that checking a donor's genetics and family history is easier compared to the first step, psychological screening. Genetic health factors are more categorical and less ambiguous. But psychological screening is much more challenging. One could argue about which factor should be number one on this list—they are both extremely important—but I (Lisa) prioritize psychological screening here because it is pointless to consider a donor's genetic history if they have not had psychological screening first. Psychological screening assesses a donor's well-being, motivation, and overall mental health. With this it may be possible to minimize the risk for future mental illness or challenges for your child-to-be.

Step 3: Undesirable Characteristics

Similarly, you may have undesirable—but not life-threatening—characteristics in your family that you do not want replicated. Think about problems that have bothered you, such as asthma or eczema. Do people in your family suffer with allergies or have the propensity for acne in their teen years? Has the genetically linked parent always disliked wearing glasses and the poor eyesight in their family? If so, take a look at the donor and their family members. Again, this is about nudging the odds in your favor, as there is no guarantee.

Compared with significant health concerns, this step may sound trivial. However, since you are choosing a donor, why not choose a donor whose family's traits you feel comfortable having in your child? Technically, three generations of information will give you the best chance of understanding which characteristics can be inherited, though many programs only provide information about the donor and her parents. While it is not ideal, looking at two generations can still be very helpful in choosing your donor.

Step 4: Open Versus Closed Donors

The world of donor conception is changing, and as we have mentioned, there is a strong trend toward openness. One day, it is likely all donors will offer some degree of openness. In the meantime, you have the option of choosing a donor who is anonymous, open, or known. These options, and the ways they may affect you and your child, are covered in chapter 5. In a nutshell, we suggest you think about how you may feel in ten to fifteen years when you may want medical information or your child is asking questions about their origins. As a parent of two donor-conceived children, I (Mark) want to help them in any way possible. Keeping the option for future contact was important for Greg and me.

Step 5: Everything Else Is Gravy

This step is *not* just a throwaway—it's the icing on the cake! From a practical point of view, if you follow the steps above, you are thoughtfully choosing the most important characteristics for your child. However, once those bases are covered, you may have some options for choosing certain characteristics you really want. For example, maybe keeping the family Italian line going or choosing a donor with a great sense of humor feels very important to you. Perhaps you really like the narrative the donor provides, and you feel their perspectives are similar to yours, or the narrative will become a nice piece of the story to tell your child. Assuming all the previous factors have been accounted for, go for it!

We talked in the previous chapter about the emotions involved in choosing a donor. While it's true—and natural—that many people feel emotional about choosing a donor, it's important not to let your emotions overwhelm your decision-making process to the point where you bypass the practical issues over which you may have some control. When my husband and I (Mark) were choosing our donor, even we found it tempting to get sidetracked by less important factors. Specifically, my partner, who is of northern European ancestry, felt that it was important to have a donor who was tall, and I, who was in tears in second grade because I had to wear glasses, wanted very much to have a donor who was not nearsighted. Those two factors represented a dream or gift we wanted to give our child, or a personal burden we wanted to relieve them of, but they complicated finding the right donor. At one point while we were laboring over our decision, we had a trusted friend at our house, and I'll never forget the moment she helped set us straight. This woman, who was five foot four with heels on, stood up on her tippy-toes, looked my husband in the eye, and said, "What's wrong with being short?"

She was right, of course, and her comment helped us remember to put nonmedical donor traits in perspective.

However, it's also true that for many people, feeling good about the donor helps them move forward. Sometimes having to use a donor may not feel so great, but imagining a desirable trait or characteristic can provide a needed sense of calm or something to feel good about. If this is you, honor your desires and make decisions that resonate with you. If you've considered all of the above and narrowed your donor options to a few promising choices, you can weigh the more emotional aspects of the decision while resting easy that you've done what you can to give yourself the healthy, happy child of your dreams.

And sometimes an emotional connection is the final piece of the puzzle that clicks into place for patients.

SAM AND JEFF

Sam immigrated to the United States from Russia with his parents and grandparents when he was young. Although they moved to a neighborhood where there were many Russian immigrants, he was an only child and spent a lot of time with his parents and grandparents. One of the activities they did together was cook. Some of his fondest memories were of making borscht and pelmeni (Russian dumplings) with his grandmother in the kitchen. Sam's partner, Jeff, on the other hand, was not very close with his parents. But Sam's family embraced Jeff, and Sam and Jeff hoped to carry Sam's family's traditions forward to future generations.

When the couple began looking for a donor, they were very focused on finding someone who was healthy and smart. They understood there was only so much control they had over the intellect of their future child, but as two successful businessmen who had attended prominent schools, they hoped to find characteristics in a donor that they would find in themselves.

However, after I (Lisa) taught them about the five-step process for choosing a donor and sketched out their priorities, those priorities began to change. As they looked through a pool of donors, sifting through health histories and looking for issues in the donors' families, they stumbled upon one donor who was special. She was a Russian immigrant whose favorite hobby was, you guessed it, cooking! They couldn't have been more excited. Unfortunately, she, like Sam, had heart disease and some other difficulties that Sam also had in his family. But she felt so perfect to them, they chose her anyway. This was not an easy decision. As practical men, they were glad to follow the plan for choosing based on family health history first, but the couple decided that if Sam were straight, he might marry someone like this and face the same challenges. Sam and Jeff had a child with this donor, and today, they are very happy.

So happy, in fact, that they decided to make their donor their friend. They hadn't married when they began treatment, and later on when they did, they invited her to their wedding. Jeff and Sam have had their donor over to cook and make Russian meals together, and she speaks Russian to their child when she sees them or they have a Zoom call. This couple decided to choose a donor who may have not been the perfect practical choice, but they thought her health history was "good enough"—and she had other qualities that, to them, made her the perfect choice.

DIANE AND DAVID

Diane, a Black woman in her midforties, and David, a Hispanic man in his late forties, came to see me (Lisa) to learn more about egg donation. We discussed options, and I provided them with an education on donor-conception issues, including disclosure and developmental issues for donor-conceived children. Both of these individuals were very successful physicians and quickly understood the importance of thinking about donor choice the way we have outlined in this book. Yet choosing a donor still felt very uncomfortable to Diane, and although she wanted to be a mother, she could not imagine how she could use the genetics of someone she didn't know to grow her family.

Then one day, Diane was having lunch with a colleague who disclosed to her that she had donated her eggs to help pay for her expenses while in medical school. Diane thought the world of this woman. She, like Diane, worked in oncology and was smart, hardworking, and dedicated to helping others. This woman was white, but Diane didn't care. She immediately started fantasizing about her colleague being her donor and couldn't wait to discuss it with David.

David was shocked. He was glad that Diane was coming around to the idea of using a donor, but he couldn't imagine having a half-Caucasian baby. He wanted to think about it and do some research to learn how it might affect the child if they did not have looks similar to Diane's. They discussed their ideas with friends who were ethicists, diversity-and-inclusion specialists, and anyone they could find who could help them make their decision. At Illume Fertility, we had many sessions to weigh the pros and cons. They had fears about how the child may feel, how they would feel, and how others may perceive their family. Fortunately, they lived in an urban area with lots of mixed-race families, which made the idea easier to accept.

The details of this story are too numerous for this space, but they did their homework, made peace with the possible ramifications of this decision, and were prepared to do all they needed to do to have a happy, healthy child and family with eggs of Diane's colleague. Diane's colleague happened to have a healthy family tree, there was no concordance of health issues, and she checked the boxes for all the things they wanted emotionally, even if those things were not what most people would expect.

Both of these couples made a decision that was based in part on emotion, but not without fully considering the practical ramifications of their decision.

USING A GESTATIONAL CARRIER

Some parents-to-be who are unable to carry a pregnancy themselves may use donated eggs and a gestational carrier. This includes single men, male same-sex couples, and women—whether single or in a relationship—who have no uterus, have uterine obstructions, or are unable to safely carry a pregnancy. For these patients, there isn't much difference in the processes of choosing a donor, the retrieval and fertilizing of eggs in the IVF laboratory, and the creation of embryos. The difference is that the embryo will be transferred to your gestational carrier with the hope of achieving a pregnancy.

When using a gestational carrier, it is important to understand that both the sperm and egg sources must be cleared by FDA regulations, which is a series of tests for sexually transmitted infections, including a physical exam and a questionnaire, which allows embryos to be cleared for transfer into a gestational carrier or surrogate. The gestational carrier should, like the donor, have proper psychological screening. However, in the interview with the gestational carrier, our assessment is different. It is less important to consider the gestational carrier's genetically linked family because you will not be using her genetics to have a child. However, if those people are part of her life, it will be very important to consider who they are, how well the family (or friendship system) functions, and how supportive they are to her and her plans to be a gestational carrier.

Many aspects of the assessment are the same or similar to the assessment for egg donors. For example, she should also have a psychological interview and a psychological test, such as the PAI or the MMPI. We also look for issues that could impact her ability to have a successful journey, such as a history of uncomplicated pregnancies, no history of untreated and unresolved traumatic experiences, no difficulty with gynecological procedures, and so on. We also want her partner to be supportive, if she has one, and ensure that she will be able to help her children understand that she will not be bringing this child home. They will not have a new brother or sister. These are only a few of the concerns to look for and discuss in the gestational carrier interview.

The gestational carrier and her partner, if she has one, should also participate in a group meeting with the intended parents. This meeting is designed to ensure that all parties have reviewed and agreed on plans for issues such as communication, spending time together socially, doctor visits, delivery plans, pumping colostrum and/or breast milk (breast-feeding is not recommended), medical testing and options regarding possibly needing to end the pregnancy prematurely, and wishes for the relationship they will have in the future. The meeting gives everyone a chance to share their feelings and work out their differences, if they have any, so we can, as we like to say, "tee everyone up for the best journey possible." The hope is that if we can address issues up front, there will be less of a chance for conflict in the future.

Moving Forward with Your Pregnancy

There's no doubt that choosing your donor is a huge, emotional decision. Some people take longer than others to grow comfortable with it, but the vast majority of people get there eventually. One thing that usually helps patients feel good is learning how the pregnancy will contribute to the development of the child. There are many ways the child will be affected by the uterine environment—the person carrying them is not just an oven! This person provides the place for the embryo to implant and the placenta for the embryo/fetus to interact with for eight months. The person who is carrying the pregnancy will provide the nutrients and help the baby grow from an embryo to a sweet bundle of joy.

There is also the process by which certain genes are turned on or off, called *epigenetics*. This is discussed in greater detail in chapter 3, but the important thing to remember is that when the egg and the sperm form an embryo, it holds many possibilities for a future person. If it develops into a baby (which not all embryos do), choices will be made. Will the child have the sperm donor's chin shape or be left-handed like their mother? Will the child have the tall stature from the egg donor's family, or will they have the athletic build of the dad's family? The environmental effects of the pregnancy in the uterus will modulate some of these features. The possibilities are too numerous to imagine. Of course, there are families where everyone is athletic or has a cleft chin, for example. But it is common to see children in a family with very different temperaments, looks, and talents. The state of the uterine environment when the baby is developing will help to turn on or off certain genes and express different traits in different people. Therefore, that baby will be uniquely yours. That child could look, sound, and behave completely differently if they were carried by someone else.

For people who carry a child conceived with the assistance of egg donation or for lesbian partners who carry a child with their partner's genetics, this can be very reassuring. For those using a gestational carrier, it may be nice to know "it takes a village," and all parties will be contributing to the development and growth of the future child.

Part III

Looking Ahead to Parenthood

8

Dealing with Practical and Ethical Dilemmas

Technology has come so far in our lifetime; we can hardly believe it. Louise Brown, the first IVF baby, was born in 1978. Her birth was proof that fertilization of an egg and a sperm outside the body was possible. The world was amazed, and more important, there was now hope for millions with infertility. Adoption was no longer the only path open to those for whom getting pregnant at home was not an option. (Unfortunately, queer and single people had fewer options because many adoption agencies would not take them in their programs. Even in the early years of IVF, few clinics would accept them.)

While IVF was a revelation for many, some people had fears about what were called at the time "test tube babies," an idea that sounded unnatural and risky to them. The media speculated that it was only a matter of time before we created "designer babies," which many worried would disrupt the natural order of things and raise myriad ethical issues. Religious groups questioned the science of IVF, suggesting that using medicine this way was ignoring God's will. These ideas, while understandable, also planted seeds of fear within the hearts and minds of people yearning to have a child. To this day, patients sometimes worry about whether they should stop treatment or not use a donor to help them build their families because if they can't get pregnant on their own, "it must not be in God's plan," even though they use medicine to help them in many other areas of their lives.

Everyone is entitled to their feelings and beliefs, and there is no one right belief system for everyone. The key is to make sure you are empowered with the facts so you can make the choice that is right for you. It's also important to understand that you are entitled to have the same dreams as others who want a family. Simply because a dream is a struggle, or takes more work than it did for your best friend, or costs more money than you would have wished, that does not mean you should not pursue it.

Perhaps most important of all is that you don't make a decision because you think you don't deserve it or because family building has been an exhausting process, and that leads you to believe that having a family is not meant for you. If you're feeling this way, we encourage you to use strategies such as those in chapter 11 to reduce your stress and emotionally reset, seek counseling so you can endure treatment, and find a way to make it happen. On the other hand, if you carefully consider all the information available to you and ultimately decide that donor-assisted conception is not for you, if it's just too much effort, time, or money, then you can stop treatment knowing you explored your options and have made a decision not only because you are feeling defeated now but because it makes sense for you and your life.

If you do decide to proceed with becoming a parent through donor conception, you will face many decisions and ethical challenges along the way. There are too many practical and ethical dilemmas to cover them all in this book, but we'll address the few that we believe will be most important to you.

Excess Embryos

As discussed in chapter 2, there is an attrition process in embryo development. When an egg and sperm are combined in a laboratory, the cells divide and eventually become a blastocyst, the stage at which there are now two types of cells making up the embryo—those of the inner cell mass, which will become the fetus, and outer cells that will eventually form the placenta. However, some embryos will not fertilize properly, and they will fail to make it to the blastocyst stage. Therefore, even though an egg donor may produce thirty eggs, it's beyond unlikely that there will be thirty embryos to use. Ten embryos might make it to the blastocyst stage, and if the recipients have those embryos screened for chromosomal abnormalities, there will likely be even fewer embryos to use.

Even so, it's common for the individual or couple to end up with more embryos than are needed to complete their family. That situation presents the parents with a dilemma—what to do with the excess embryos. They can choose to discard them, donate them to science, or donate them to another individual or couple. It can be very difficult to be faced with this decision. Discarding embryos can feel harsh, particularly when you have children at home who were conceived with the same batch of embryos. People often look at their children and think of those embryos as would-be siblings, even though, according to science, this is not truly the case. Regardless, many patients feel paralyzed by this decision and end up leaving unused embryos in storage for years to put off making it.

As families hold on to their embryos and kick the metaphorical can down the road, storage fees continue to accumulate, and eventually, the family will decide to close that chapter and plan for the disposition of their embryos. Since it's unlikely to have a child by accident, making the decision about what to do with the remaining embryos means accepting that there will be no more children. This can feel quite sad. It can also be a source of conflict if the parents in a couple have different feelings about having another child, and especially upsetting for the partner who had hoped for a larger family. Patients are often surprised how frequently they have feelings of grief or loss when they dispose of their embryos.

Let's go through your options one at a time. If you're in the early stages of your journey with donor-assisted conception, this decision may feel like it is too far in the future to worry about now, but it's helpful to understand your choices and start thinking about them so that you will be more prepared later.

Discarding Embryos

Discarding embryos can take many forms. Some people choose to have the clinic discard the embryos, meaning there is no continued intervention to keep them possibly viable (and we say *possibly* because it is impossible to predict which embryos could have created a healthy baby). For many, this choice makes the most sense. If you do not wish to use them or donate them to science, deciding to no longer intervene to keep them possibly viable could be the right choice for you.

I (Lisa) have helped patients create ceremonies where they write a letter to the dream or fantasy of the child they may have had and burn the paper. Some people will take home the small test tubes (called *pipettes*), which have been opened and exposed to air so that they will no longer be viable. They may want to bury the pipette and plant a tree in its place. Rituals and ceremonies can be helpful to some, as they can help close that chapter in their lives and pay homage to the fertility journey, the hardships they have endured, and the children they will not create.

Donating Embryos to Science

When embryos are donated to science, they are often used to help the scientists practice their craft. These embryos can be used to change the way we scientifically evaluate embryos for their competency and potential success to help people have children in the future. Many people find comfort in this option because it feels like they are giving back to the science that has made their family possible. They may want to "pay it forward" and contribute to a younger generation of scientists who may help advance the technology and therefore benefit the lives of many yearning to have children.

However, this is not an attractive option for some. Some believe that science should only be used to create life, or they do not like the idea of science interfering with their embryos. Sometimes these ideas come from an emotional place or from a religious perspective.

Donating to Others

Some patients prefer to donate their surplus embryos to others who want to build a family. For some who have completed their family, donating unused embryos to other people through an embryo donation group feels good. They know how hard the process is, and they are happy to help others see their dreams of building a family come true.

What does it mean to those patients, those parents-to-be who choose to use donated embryos? It can be a wonderful option, and not dissimilar to using donated sperm or eggs. It is less expensive than using an egg donor or a sperm donor because the embryos are free—they were *donated*—and typically patients only need to pay for basic medical procedures and the costs of transferring the embryo to the uterus. We have worked with many people who could not otherwise afford to build their families. Fertility treatment can be extremely expensive, and by the time people have experienced repeated failed attempts to become pregnant, they are drained both emotionally and financially. Thus, the process of embryo donation can be a win-win—the donors feel good about giving their embryos to a family whose lives they will change forever, and the recipients finally have the opportunity to parent. Many of our patients who use donated embryos report that they feel a boost of confidence knowing the embryos they receive come from a batch that already created one or more children. These recipients also often feel the embryo donation process is emotionally fulfilling because the embryos were created from love.

On the other hand, many potential embryo donors never get past the emotional hurdle that someone else will be raising a genetically linked brother or sister to their own child or children.

If you are planning to donate your embryos, some of the questions you may want to ask yourself are:

- Do you want to have an open relationship with the recipients of your embryos? If so, what would that look like?

- Would the children be friends or regard themselves as siblings?
- What if there is a rift in the relationship you have with the parents of that child?
- Can you see that child as their child and not yours?
- If you do not want to have an open relationship, can you accept that it will be important for your child to know about the siblings?
- Can you feel at peace knowing that child is "out there" and not feel preoccupied with where they are and if you will see them in the supermarket one day?

There are many issues to consider, and again, there is no right answer—just the right answer for you and your family.

DONATING TO AN EMBRYO ADOPTION GROUP

Embryo adoption is different from embryo donation in one important way. Embryo adoption typically involves a standard adoption process, including detailed paperwork and a home study. The organizations that run these programs often only accept Christian heterosexual couples and generally request that they raise the child Christian. A couple undergoing embryo adoption is likely agreeing that they are adopting the embryo/person. According to the scientific point of view, the embryo is not yet a person. It can have many uses in addition to creating a child, but it is not a child. The American Society for Reproductive Medicine and other groups have addressed this issue, and many in the field of reproductive medicine have concerns about embryo adoption.

It is important to understand this before donating to an embryo adoption group. For heterosexual Christian couples who believe that the embryo is a person, donating your surplus embryos to an embryo adoption group could be a good option. For others, it conflicts with their value system. As with so many of the issues in the chapter, there is no right answer—just the right answer for you. The important element in all these decisions is to be educated.

One final note about embryo donation. Although it can be a positive and fulfilling option for patients with excess embryos, and it can be a great way for prospective parents to build their family, it is not a perfect process from the recipient's point of view. There are two common issues for concern. First, many (but not all) embryo donation programs are designed to be anonymous, and this can be stressful for families who would like an open relationship with their donors. Second, depending on the program, the embryo donors may or may not have had the same rigorous screening process that an anonymous sperm or egg donor may have had. Many programs believe that requiring embryo donors to go through multiple medical and psychological hurdles to donate may pose too much of an obstacle for those donors and that they may be less inclined to donate their embryos as a result. Some embryos have had genetic testing, and others have not. If the person donating used a donor, you may have additional information and the assurance that one of the donors had psychological testing. However, this is not the case for all embryos. Some embryos are simply donated from a heterosexual couple who froze embryos with their own gametes created with IVF. Genetic testing will help families who use these donors discover information about their children, and the science is improving every day, but not all embryos are tested. So, some embryos may have more detailed information than others, and therefore accepting some embryos may require taking a bigger leap of faith than others.

Compassionate Transfers

While this is not an option used by many, we have found that it is important for patients to know about because some people decide it is the only option right for them. It is possible for your doctor to transfer an embryo into the vagina at a time that it is unlikely you or the person carrying will become pregnant. For people who desire to leave as much as possible up to God or fate, a compassionate transfer is a helpful choice. For people who are religious or have ethical struggles with the other options, this choice offers an opportunity to not deliberately discard their embryos and allow them to pass within their body.

Screening for Heritable Diseases

As we have discussed, not only will your donor be screened for genetic disorders related to disease but so will the parent(s)-to-be who are genetically linked to the embryo. The purpose of this, of course, is to increase your chances of having a successful pregnancy and a healthy child. But if thinking about potential risks for your future child was not stressful enough, you can probably see why this might be stressful for another reason. Any risks revealed in the screening are, inherently, risks to the genetically linked parent-to-be who was tested. If screening identifies some-thing that could possibly affect your health (for example, if you discover you are positive for BRCA, the breast cancer gene), it could be valuable information, as it may help you act on possible preventative measures. At the same time, it can be difficult to learn that you are potentially at risk for any disease, particularly one that can be life-threatening, such as Huntington's disease. If you receive unwanted news about your genetics, you may want to seek support from a professional who understands your unique hardship. Many clinics employ or have access to mental health profession-als who can help you manage stress stemming from the diagnosis and also help you with decision-making related to future treatments or testing.

We have met some patients who prefer not to know. Sometimes they have a fear of a particular issue. In rare cases, there is a heritable family difficulty that the patient may or may not have contracted. Sometimes knowing about that difficulty can change their quality of life, and they decide they would rather not know. Only a minority of patients decline this testing, but it is an option that you have every right to exercise.

Dealing with Egg and Sperm Problems

When patients learn of a diagnosis of a problem with their sperm or eggs, they can feel like a tidal wave has hit them. They may feel shock, anger, and disbelief, and the diagnosis may take some time to absorb. However, because eggs and sperm are very different cells, the paths forward from these two diagnoses are different. Typically, when a difficulty with your eggs is discovered, your doctor will likely suggest donor eggs as the next best option. In contrast, there are multiple issues that can present a difficulty for the sperm, and many of these issues can be resolved.

Some sperm issues are major, such as when there is no sperm or the sperm cannot be used at all. In these cases, a sperm donor is probably the best solution. Other problems with sperm, while significant, can be addressed with medication, a small procedure, or even a surgery to attempt to extract viable sperm. Even though we have options, the solutions are not necessarily a slam dunk. The medications prescribed can cause reactions, the medical procedures can be uncomfortable, and, for some, the process of the doctor appointments and procedures can feel upsetting and emotionally diminishing. Many prefer to endure these treatments to have a genetically connected child, but many don't, and you will want to get good counsel and think carefully about your options if you have a sperm difficulty.

It's important not to minimize the impact a sperm difficulty can have on the patient or the couple. There tends to be a great deal of focus on women's difficulty when their egg quality diminishes, but men can also feel the hurt and grief of not being able to use their genetics to build a family. They also may feel its effect on their sense of self as a man and their vision of how they would become a father. They may feel deeply affected by the loss of a genetic tie to their future child or the loss of familial connection to their ancestors and more. For many, these losses can feel huge, and they need to be worked through. Addressing them can not only help the person struggling but also be of enormous help to the couple.

Sometimes the patient who is diagnosed with a gamete problem has less difficulty accepting the news than their partner. Not being able to conceive using the sperm or eggs of the one you love can feel deeply unfair, and sometimes the unaffected partner feels it would be impossible to imagine using donor gametes to have a child. Some may have the perspective that they partnered with this person to build a family with them and did not sign up to use donor genetics. It can feel impossible for these people to move forward with treatment. It is essential for that person and for the couple to seek counseling to manage the stress and keep the relationship intact.

Embryo Screening
(Preimplantation Genetic Testing)

We discussed preimplantation genetic testing, a technique to screen for genetically linked difficulties in embryos, on page 69. For some patients, the thought of using PGT is a no-brainer. For others, it's a needless expense. And for still others, it can also feel like using this technology is crossing an ethical or religious line. Wherever you stand on the issue, there are some dilemmas to consider.

First, while embryo screening provides obvious advantages toward improving your chances of having a healthy pregnancy and ultimately a healthy child, there are some downsides. Here are a few:

- Embryo screening can be expensive.
- Embryo screening does not guarantee that children will be healthy or free of birth defects and learning differences.
- Embryo screening is not a perfect science, and the question of whether an embryo is viable is not always a black-and-white matter. Some imperfect embryos could possibly create a healthy child (though it may be a slim possibility). When embryos fall in a gray area, the scientist needs to make a judgment call, and as a result, there may be embryos that could have been viable that will not be approved for transfer.

- Embryo screening is a physical process of microscopic surgery and runs the risk of damaging an otherwise healthy embryo 1–3 percent of the time.
- Some people, for religious or ethical reasons, do not feel comfortable with the idea of testing an embryo.

PGT-A refers to screening embryos specifically for aneuploidy, meaning one or more of the chromosomes are abnormal. It is important to know that, at the time of this writing, PGT-A screens for many difficulties but does not screen for everything—for example, for autism, birth defects, or developmental delays. Genetic counselors often see patients shocked when a transfer of a normal embryo does not work or, even more stressful, when a child is born with a birth defect. This can lead to great stress and disappointment in parents when they believed they had done everything they could and something else (nonchromosomal) is wrong with their child. PGT-A moves the needle to a healthier child but in no way provides a guarantee. However, since numerical chromosome abnormalities are present in 30–80 percent of embryos (depending on the age of the egg source) and are the reason for more than 50 percent of miscarriages, PGT-A does provide a great deal of information.

If you're using an egg donor or if you have young eggs, you have a much better chance of having healthy embryos than if you used the eggs of a woman who is over thirty-five years of age when she had her eggs retrieved. Although many of our patients opt to use this technology with donor eggs, which are typically young, in these cases, PGT-A does not always feel as necessary.

Another possible advantage—or possible dilemma—to screening embryos is that the screening will reveal the sex of the embryos. Then the patient is left with the decision about which embryos to transfer. Some programs will readily offer patients this option, but others feel more strongly that the screening should be based on health rather than the preference of the sex of the future child. Knowing the sex of the embryo before there is an ongoing pregnancy can bring up a host of issues for the patient. For example, they may have fantasies about the girl or boy they will have, and what if that embryo does not result in a successful pregnancy? Or worse, what if there is a loss? They may think about that boy or girl in more intense detail than they would have if they hadn't known the sex, and it may cause more upset. They tend to feel as if they lost their "little girl" or "little boy," not just that they lost the pregnancy. Personalizing the embryo very early on, especially if there is not another embryo of the desired sex available, can be devastating for some parents-to-be.

The healthiest or most cellular embryos have the greatest chance of leading to an ongoing pregnancy, but sometimes the embryo of the desired sex is not the embryo that is the healthiest. When that happens, the intended parent or parents are forced to decide between transferring the "best" embryo or the embryo of their preferred sex. We have seen many instances when the parents don't agree on this decision, but most agree to transfer the healthiest embryo first.

Later, they may return to the clinic and choose the next healthiest embryo or the other sex for family balancing.

When parents-to-be are very focused on the sex of their future child, we encourage them to remember that in our modern world, many of our old, preconceived notions associated with sex are no longer wholly valid. The desire to have a girl to take care of you when you are older, for example, or a boy to carry on the family name are more romanticized images than they are likely realities for a child born in the twenty-first century. As a gay man, I (Mark) never met my parents' expectations of marrying a woman, but I was able to "give" them grandchildren. It's important to understand that your future child may not fit into historical gender roles.

We have also seen situations where inheritance may be involved, or where the specific culture of the patient has led them to desire one sex over the other. In our decades of experience, we have seen many complex situations, and we would not presume that we know every person's unique circumstance. But overall, we believe that patients have the right to know the sex of their embryo, though they need to be counseled strongly. Once you know the sex of the embryo, it's not something a patient can unknow. Some see the fertility journey as being very planned and scientific, and not knowing the sex of their future child is a way to have one surprise on their road to parenthood. We agree, and we believe parents will love any child they have and, for some couples, knowing the sex can create unnecessary stress in the relationship.

Dilemmas Faced by LGBTQIA+ Patients

From 2014 to 2017, embryo transfers to gestational carriers increased 146 percent. According to the Society for Assisted Reproductive Technology, 48 percent of those were for male intended fathers in 2017. This timing seems to correspond with the legalization of gay/queer marriage in the United States. At the time of writing, greater than 60 percent of transfers into a gestational carrier are linked to male intended parents.

Our practice is fully inclusive, and we are a Healthcare Equality Leader as per the Human Rights Campaign. With this designation, we have become a safe and welcoming place for the LGBTQIA+ community. We have had the honor and privilege of working with thousands of people across the rainbow of our community. And we have seen a steep increase in patients seeking care. This is great news. As a dad through egg donation and surrogacy and a member of the community, it is my (Mark's) personal passion to help everyone navigate the complex issue of family building. I am regularly amazed by couples I see who are in their twenties and have been together for five to ten years and are getting married and having kids. So many walls have come down, and it is simply wonderful to witness. We are thrilled that more and more queer couples feel comfortable and empowered to have the families of their dreams.

Unfortunately, many insurance plans do not cover fertility treatment for queer couples. We hope to see this change, but until then, it means the cost for LGBTQIA+ parenthood can be completely out of pocket. For some, it can run into the hundreds of thousands of dollars. Some people decide to have fewer children as a way to cut costs by not pursuing some treatments. Others borrow, save, or get a second mortgage to have a child. These decisions need to be made with your partner, if you have one, and perhaps with a financial counselor to help you plan for the decisions that are coming your way.

Besides how to pay for treatment, queer couples assigned male at birth are faced with other specific dilemmas. To begin, do they use the genetics of both partners as sperm sources or one? In 2019, we published research that found that the majority of male couples we see desire to have a child from each of their genetics.[1] Since these men will also need a surrogate to have a child, and each surrogacy journey can cost $200,000 or more, many men will request that their doctor use an embryo created from each partner and that the surrogate will carry twins.

While this is completely understandable, it is not the safest decision. The American Society for Reproductive Medicine (2021) issued guidelines[2] for clinics to transfer only one embryo at a time in patients with the highest chance for pregnancy. This decision was based on convincing evidence for the increased risk of complications (including some that could be life-threatening) for the babies and/or the person carrying the multiple pregnancy. Once our dads-to-be understand this, they usually decide to have one child at a time. However, this means they will need to spend the money for two surrogacy journeys or decide to have just one child with the sperm of one partner. How will they choose?

Sometimes one partner's preference to use his genetics is stronger than the other partner's, so the couple will use the sperm of the man who feels more strongly about it. Perhaps one partner has nieces and nephews and sees his "genetic legacy" continue in his extended family, so he does not feel the same need to reproduce with his genetics. In some cases, one partner may have medical or psychiatric issues in his family that he does not want to see continue in his future child, so he decides not to use his genetics. These discussions are complicated and highly personal, as you can see in the following story.

RON AND LUKE

Although they were not fully educated on how to choose a donor or the surrogacy process, Ron and Luke came to us already having witnessed several of their same-sex male friends go through their family-building journeys, and they were more prepared than most. They had planned for the time the process would take, the amount of money it would cost, and some of the challenges they may face along the way. In addition, they both had strong support networks. Their parents, siblings, and friends were excited for them and couldn't wait to hear about the details of their journey.

Ron and Luke planned to use both of their

sperm to fertilize eggs and planned to have a child with each of their genetics. They both beamed with excitement as they told me (Lisa) their plan. In their vision, an embryo created with Ron's sperm would be used for baby number one, and an embryo created with Luke's sperm would be used for baby number two. "Actually, neither one of us has a strong preference for which embryo will go first," Luke explained. "How we decided was—my two sisters already have children, and I am a big part of their lives, and plus, that helps Mom and Dad feel a bit less eager, you know? But Ron is an only child." He put a hand on Ron's knee. "So, since I have already been able to see my family's genetics on the faces of little people, we thought Ron should go first."

Unfortunately, it did not work out as planned. There was no sperm in Ron's semen. They consulted with a urologist who suggested hormones and a surgical procedure to extract sperm. Nothing worked. This eager, earnest couple was now distraught. Some friends and family members suggested Ron use a cousin's sperm, but the two men understood how complicated that may be and decided against it. Eventually, they decided to have children with embryos created with Luke's sperm only. Although Ron felt that any children created with either of their sperm would be their children together, he also tearfully admitted that not being able to have a child with his genetics felt like a personal wound. He was sure he would recover, but at the time, it did feel hurtful.

Ron and Luke are very happy now with their family of four and wouldn't change it for the world.

Some couples fertilize eggs with both of their sperm and plan for one child, with the hope they may one day be able to return to the clinic to undergo another gestational carrier journey with the other partner's sperm. Others are able to use a family member as a donor so they can have genetics from both families. Until financial reimbursement for queer families is the norm, this will continue to be a dilemma faced by gay male couples who use donor conception to build their families.[3] As with so many things on the donor-conception journey, it's very important to discuss such issues not only with each other but also with your doctor and a counselor.

Lesbian women face some similar difficulties but also need to consider others. They need to decide who will use their genetics and who will carry the pregnancy. In our preliminary research, we are finding that some women prefer to carry, some prefer to use their genetics, and some don't have a preference.[4] It is also possible for each partner to carry an embryo created with the other partner's egg. This is called *reciprocal IVF* and is a wonderful but more expensive way both partners can share in the pregnancy.

Another option for lesbian couples is to use INVOcell, a

product that allows the sperm and egg to be fertilized, placed in a small container, and inserted into one of the partners. This process can help each partner to feel involved and also can reduce the cost of treatment because the lab does not need to be as involved in culturing sperm, egg, and embryo. Choosing it can be a dilemma, though, because the procedure is not as effective as IVF. It is important to weigh the benefits, costs, and chances for success with your doctor and counselor.

One of the most important issues to be aware of if you are a same-sex female couple is your age. It's not fair, and it is upsetting to think about it, but, as one of our favorite *Star Wars* characters may have said if he worked in reproductive medicine, "Think about it, you must." In our experience, reproductive aging in women remains the most significant hurdle to get past irrespective of sexuality. Many women who are thirty-eight and above have lost a great deal of fertility potential—that is, they have very few good eggs left. One of our goals in writing this book is to help people prevent regrets, and this is a place where a little forward thinking could prevent a lot of regret.

Consider this scenario: You are thirty-two, and your partner is thirty-five. You have a strong desire to carry and use your genetics, while your partner doesn't feel as strongly about either. Since you want to carry and use your genetics, you start with IUI. It's less expensive than IVF, and your doctor tells you that the odds are in your favor for a healthy pregnancy. You become pregnant and have a baby. Parenting is better than either of you could have anticipated, and your partner's feelings have changed—she would like to try next. However, more than three years have passed since you both began treatment, and she is now thirty-eight and has difficulty becoming pregnant.

What can you do to change this outcome? Your partner could go first, but in this imaginary scenario, that is not what you or your partner wanted. Another option is that your partner could undergo IVF at the same time as you and create embryos with the same sperm you are using. In that situation, you would attempt pregnancy and she would freeze her embryos. Now, when you return for baby number two, her embryos are thirty-five instead of thirty-eight, and that can make a big difference for women trying to become pregnant. Fertility preservation can allow a woman to "stop the clock." It is not a guarantee of future success, but it can dramatically increase your odds of having that second child, minimize your risk for miscarriage, and give you both a chance to breathe and enjoy baby number one a little more because you won't feel like you are racing with the clock.

Dilemmas Faced by Single Parents-to-Be

Single parenthood was considered shameful for many years. It was 1981 when single mother-to-be Jane Mattes decided she needed support from other women facing the same struggles she was and began her support organization, Single Mothers by Choice. Since then, the organization has grown to more than thirty thousand members. Today, many fertility organizations, fertility clinics, and therapy programs have single-mother support programs, and more and more single fathers are choosing to parent alone as well. We have seen this in our practice, where an increasing number of single parents-to-be create families—whether they are men or women, straight or LGBTQIA+. Some decide to co-parent with a friend. Others decide that their support network is sufficient, they have the finances to care for a child, and they do not want to wait for the right partner.

Clearly, the face of the modern family is changing. Today, with so many celebrities becoming single parents, instead of being shameful, single parenting is practically fashionable. However, it still presents challenges. As a single parent-to-be, you may face most of the dilemmas discussed in this chapter, but you will face those decisions without a partner. That may be difficult. It also may be difficult to endure treatment, be pregnant, give birth, and manage a home, career, and the daily tasks of child-rearing alone. Does this mean it shouldn't be done? No. But if you decide to parent alone, it is very important to fully embrace it. You can gain help from a knowledgeable counselor and shore up your support systems so you can prepare yourself for the road ahead.

Many people still think about marriage as coming before the baby carriage, as the rhyme goes. Yet that is changing. We see many people who start out as single parents who later meet someone who does or doesn't have children, and then they parent together. In today's world, many options are possible, and we encourage you to feel confident that many options are possible for you as well.

"It Doesn't Feel Good to Use Eggs/Sperm from Someone Who Sold Their Gametes"

We are glad you brought this up. Many people are upset not knowing the motivation of the donor, and we are happy to dispel the myths. We have some insight from our friends at sperm banks and from the counselors who screen sperm donors, but most of our understanding of donors' motivations comes from the egg donors we see every week (and we have seen thousands). Many of their motives are the same: They would like to help a couple or individual have a child. Are they interested in the compensation they will receive? Yes, but that is only part of their motivation. To pass psychological screening and be selected as a donor, they also need to have an altruistic motivation.

The stories we hear from egg donors often fall into three categories. The first are women who are single and pursuing a career. They want to pay off student debt or could use a little financial help to pay for living expenses while they are in school. A second group is women who say that they do not plan to have children but that they want to put their eggs, and good genetics, to use to help someone who does want children. We may advise some of these women to freeze eggs for themselves, because when they are in their thirties, they may change their mind. Egg freezing is certainly not a guarantee, but we want the donors to understand that if they decide later in life to have children of their own and then need donor eggs themselves, that could be devastating for them. Last, we see women who had children at a fairly young age and do not desire more children. They adore their children and love being mothers. These women often say that they cannot imagine what it would be like to not be able to have a child and would like to help a couple or individual achieve their dreams.

This is only a short list of the quandaries we see people face as they move through reproductive medicine and donor conception to have a child. One dilemma we haven't talked about in this chapter is a topic that every parent-to-be of a donor-conceived child will face—disclosure. Some parents feel the decision to disclose to their future child is very easy, some find that decision very difficult, and still others are somewhere in between. Many are troubled by the questions of how or when to disclose. And many parents, plenty occupied with the immediate challenges and dilemmas of the donor-conception journey, simply put off the topic for later consideration. But as you will see, this is a topic for right now. Even if you are only considering donor conception, it's important to know what you're signing up for, what will be important for your future child, and how to begin to set the wheels in motion for your future right now.

9

Disclosure

*What Your Child Needs to Know (And Why
It's Helpful to Start Practicing Now)*

The topic of disclosing information to future children raises anxiety for many parents-to-be of donor-conceived children. For some patients, it can even be so distressing that it prevents them from moving forward in treatment. Patients worry that their child will not understand donor conception or reject them once they do understand. It is our hope that this chapter will allay some of those fears while also providing you with best practices for talking to donor-conceived children about how they came into your family and helping you understand why it's important to begin to think about this early on. While nothing in your past could have prepared or educated you for this future conversation, you can gain confidence with education and preparation.

Why Disclose?

As you read this, you may be feeling like disclosure is just too much for you to deal with; perhaps you have even considered not telling. Here are a few reasons why we strongly urge you not to avoid disclosing to your child.

First, as discussed in chapter 5, there is no such thing as anonymity. Your child will discover their origins at some point. If you have told anyone along the way, the secret can leak out. Inexpensive at-home genetic testing can quickly uncover the truth about who we are and are not genetically related to, and many schools are assigning genetic testing homework as part of the biology curriculum. A child can also learn about their origins through an accidental discovery on the internet or by learning the truth of their origins under difficult circumstances. For example, I (Lisa) once worked with a woman who used ovum donation to have her children and later developed breast cancer. She discovered she was BRCA positive. Her daughter was distraught about her mother's diagnosis, but she also naturally worried that she too was BRCA positive. It was the worst possible time to disclose to her daughter, who had to deal with the upset of her mother's diagnosis and, at the same time, learn that she was not genetically connected to her. For this young woman, it was devastating. She felt lied to, which affected her relationship with her mother, and she struggled to re-calibrate her identity. She thought she was like her mother in so many ways, and although these things did not change, she had to realize it wasn't about their genetic link. Some people adjust to their new identity more easily than others. For this woman, it was an extremely difficult revelation during an extremely difficult time. There are many accounts of donor-conceived adults saying that learning later in life has caused an identity crisis for them—they thought they knew who they were their whole lives and then discovered their genetic makeup was totally different. We feel that the child has a right to know. Even if you don't agree, keep in mind that you will not be able to guarantee anonymity.

Once you have your child, you will live a life like everyone else. Your days will be filled with changing diapers, packing school lunches, and taking your child to music lessons. However, it's possible that not telling (or holding in a secret) may create a negative feeling internally, which can cause you discomfort and also unconsciously be communicated to your children. In one study, mothers who did not tell their children experienced fewer positive interactions with their children than women who conceived with their own gametes.[1] It has also been shown that parents who disclose experience less stress and anxiety,[2] and, for parents who disclose before the age of seven, research demonstrates higher levels of adolescent well-being and more positive family relationships.[3]

Another consideration is consanguinity, or having a genetic connection to someone you become romantically or sexually involved with. While it is not common, it does happen, and probably more often than we suspect. We know of a case from several years ago when two families underwent fertility treatment at a fertility clinic in a small town. The families used the same egg donor. By sheer coincidence, they also used the same sperm donor. These children do not know they are full genetic siblings and are being raised in the same small town. They are probably in school together and may even play on the same sports teams.

If your child is donor-conceived and they meet someone they like, they should feel empowered and educated to ask that person if they were donor-conceived, or if their parent was a donor. If the other child says yes, they can easily use a commercial DNA testing program to identify if they are genetically related. Another possibility is that one of their parents was an egg donor or sperm donor, and therefore they are related through that parent's donation event. I (Lisa) share this information with all the donors I screen because their children (and their siblings' children) are also at risk. There's no way around it. This is the new reality in our world, and it's an important reason for making sure your child knows they were conceived with the help of a donor.

How can this happen? While the American Society for Reproductive Medicine has issued guidelines about how often someone should donate, there is no national enforcement of those guidelines in the United States. An egg donor may donate a few times to a clinic, and the clinic will likely limit their donations and not allow them to continue to donate beyond the number recommended by the ASRM. The donor can agree but later change her mind or go to another clinic, agency, or online donor program. Each of those donations can result in several offspring. She can also donate to an egg bank. Young women can make twenty or more eggs, and because egg banks often sell them in lots of six, there is an increased likelihood that most of her eggs will be used to produce children. Likewise, a sperm donor can "retire" from a sperm bank and then donate to many more sperm banks. They can also donate to friends or donate to someone online. We are beginning to see more and more people find each other online.

Embryo donation can further increase the odds of meeting a genetic relative. As we have discussed, a family with excess embryos can donate them to science, dispose of them, or donate them to another family. The donation can happen through their clinic or through an embryo donation program. At our program, we once worked with a woman who donated seven embryos to seven families around the country. Therefore, in addition to the offspring created by the families who used gamete donation, there may be more families receiving unused embryos, creating more children in more families.

It's also not possible to know how old your child's donor-conceived siblings will be. As far as we know, there is no limit on the length of time you can store your embryos. Currently, there are many embryos that have been frozen for decades, and there has already been one child born from a twenty-seven-year-old embryo.[4] This means your child will not only likely have many donor siblings, but some can be decades younger than your child, so your child's children will need to be aware of this as well.

We are not sharing this to shock or worry you. It's a matter of learning to accept this reality so you can inform your children and move into this new, and still unregulated, world in which we live. We can all learn to accept it, just as we have accepted other confusing or difficult things in life. Some people worry that these issues will prevent them from living a "normal life." You deserve to enjoy parenthood to its fullest, and you can, but if you plan to have donor-conceived children, these are new realities that are important to understand.

Why Start Early?

So, if we decide to tell our children, when should we do it? Our strong advice is to start early—ideally when they are in the crib. To understand why, consider two important points that professionals in the adoption community have made—points that also relate to gamete donation. First, many people who have nongenetically related children have some discomfort about how they built their family. If they experienced fertility treatment, discussing their journey may also trigger painful memories. If they are part of a same-sex couple, they will need to explain where the other gametes came from. If they are a single parent, they need to explain why there is one parent instead of two. In any of these scenarios, parents can be nervous. How can they explain such complicated information to a young child? Will they get it right? Will their child have good self-esteem and feel close to them?

If a parent is nervous, they may stumble over their words when talking with their children about their beginnings. If the child sees their parents appear nervous when talking to them about the way they were conceived, it's unlikely they will think, *My parents love me, and they are just trying to get this right.* They are more likely to think, *If the way my family was built is not a problem, why are my parents acting so weird around this topic?!*

Starting early helps you avoid that. If you speak to your children from day one, before the child can understand what is being said, you have the opportunity to craft a narrative that feels comfortable, work it through with your partner, and then work out the kinks as you rehearse your story over and over. You can stumble over your words, you can have your tears, you and your partner, if you have one, can disagree and modify your narrative, and eventually, after reworking your story and then practicing that story, you will become more comfortable, and the narrative will eventually roll off your tongue easily. When your little one is old enough to understand what you're saying, the child has heard it many times, and it's likely to feel very natural. It will be part of the backdrop of their lives. That is certainly the case in both of our homes, where our children learned of their stories from day one.

Adoption and donor conception are different in many ways, but in many ways, they are also similar. One of the lessons we have learned from the adoption community is that early disclosure can be helpful for children and for their parents.[5] Experts have argued that disclosure is not a onetime event but a process of sharing the story over time, thereby creating a comfortable and natural atmosphere where the adoption story is simply part of the *family* story. Many adult adoptees say they appreciate having "always known" rather than being told as a single event. This idea of starting early and "dropping seeds" over time is becoming more widely accepted in the donor-conception community as well. These seeds can be dropped throughout the child's childhood. One way to do this is through metaphors. For example, when playing with a toy truck, you might talk about parts. "This is a Toyota truck, but it has a Ferrari engine. Sometimes all our parts come from our family, and sometimes some of our parts come from other people." There are a lot of ways to bring up the subject over time to help normalize it for your child and convey a sense of acceptance and warmth for your donor, which will, by extension, eventually be valued by your child. Remember, even if your child is just like you in every way imaginable—they like bike riding like you, they love eating pizza on Sunday nights like you, and they even have the same sense of humor— part of them is connected to someone else in the world, and they need to know that you feel good about all of them, not only the parts that are connected to you.

One important note: While it's never too early to begin

disclosing to your child, it's also never too late, so if you have a donor-conceived child and have not disclosed yet, being angry with yourself about it won't help. I (Lisa) have helped many families disclose to their child later. The important thing is that you tell, and find a way to tell that you can feel good about, so your child will hear the information in a warm and positive manner.

BRING IN THE BOOKS

It can also be helpful to use books that speak about the child's beginning in different ways. You can find books that discuss the donor-conception story in a narrative form, in more technical terms, or in metaphor. Find some books that work for you and your family, and read them with your child. As you go through these books, find pieces that speak to you, and spend extra time on those parts. You can modify stories in ways that make sense for you and your partner, if you have one. This way you can feel a sense of investment and ownership over your story. You can find a regularly updated list of recommended books at the website for the Center for Family Building: www.familybuilding.net.

It's also nice for the child to have a book of their own—a book that tells *their* story. Lifebooks have been popular in the adoption community for decades, and we recommend them for donor-conceived families as well. The next chapter explains how to make a lifebook and when to start (hint: now!).

Research supports the idea that telling earlier can be more helpful to the offspring and to their relationship with their parents.[6] A recent study found that donor-conceived people "were more likely to have positive feelings surrounding their conception if they are told at a young age by a family member and have regularly updated and accessible medical information."[7]

There has been discussion, and research, about donor-conceived children who are a bit older. Some professionals felt that talking to your child when they begin school made sense. It's been argued that this is a time they begin to understand biology. Their friends may be gaining second or third siblings, and it's common for children to have questions about why, for instance, Sammy's mom has a big belly. This is a natural time to have a conversation about the birds and the bees and maybe raise the concept of a donor. You may want to say, "Yes, Sammy's mom is having a baby. Do you know you need three things to have a baby? A sperm, an egg, and a uterus? We have two (or one or don't have any) of those things, so we found a wonderful doctor/agency/lawyer who introduced us to this nice woman (or man), and they helped us have you."

Many parents-to-be of donor-conceived children have a negative reaction to the idea of talking to their young child about their donor story. For one thing, they wonder how a child will understand something so complex at such a young age. We often hear comments such as, "I don't want to confuse my child until they can understand," or "I don't want them to feel different," or "I don't want their friends to think they are different." Some fear that when the child learns they do not have a genetic tie to the parent, they will reject the parent or regard the donor as the parent. Or they worry that somehow being open about their child's origins will change the dynamic in the family. Their family will not be like other families. What research has shown, however, is that although the difference is small, children can feel a greater sense of cohesiveness with their parents when they learn when they are very young.[8]

The truth is, your family *won't* be the same as other families, but all families are different. And that's not a bad thing. It's something to get used to, it's something you will need to incorporate into your life, and it will, believe it or not, be something that you can embrace. When you embark on your donor-conception journey, your thoughts about your donor may be front and center in your mind. That feeling may make you uneasy, feeling like the child will be different from you since they will be related to someone you may not know. But you will love your child, and your child will love you. You will love the way they look, the funny giggles they have, and how they may squint when they smile. That child will depend on you and will look at you with adoration in their eyes. When these things happen, you are likely to feel very grateful to that person who helped you create your family. Once you feel these feelings, you'll likely want to do all you can to honor them and perhaps even connect with them and/or donor-related siblings.

Many years ago, there was some discussion about how to decorate your home with Chinese artifacts if you had adopted a child from China. Some people suggested that the child's room should have the Chinese artifacts, while others said only the communal living spaces should have artifacts, which would be "decorations" in the home. The experts weighed in, and the answer was to have Chinese artifacts throughout the home because that family is now a Chinese American family. It's not just a home with parents and children. Everyone is on the same team, and everyone embraces one another. Likewise, your family will become a family created by donor conception. We're not suggesting that you should decorate your home with pictures of your donor everywhere. What we're saying is that although it may feel impossible in the beginning, you can grow and become comfortable being a family created by donor conception.

Being open with your child from the beginning, or as young as possible, caring about the things that they may care about as they grow, and fostering a close and connected family is the goal. A study conducted with offspring created with sperm donation found that "adolescents who were securely attached to their mothers were more accepting of their donor conception than insecurely attached adolescents, suggesting that quality of mother-child relationships influences feelings about donor conception."[9] Therefore, building a close relationship where your child can feel good about themselves and close to you can help your child at many stages of their lives, and being their ally in their self-discovery will be one more gift you can give them as a parent.

I (Lisa) see many parents and parents-to-be who are concerned that their children will be upset with them for using donor conception. They also worry that the children will feel upset or "different" if they know they were donor-conceived. One day, donor conception will be seen as "normal," but until then, it is true that it's still considered "different" by many. As more people from all kinds of families discuss the way their families were built, donor conception will become more familiar. This is similar to the way adoption evolved. Adult children spoke openly about their feelings about being adopted, and the stigma began to shrink. The rise of single parents, LGBTQIA+ parents, and open donor relationships has also helped change the ways people are defining the word *family*.

You don't know how your child will feel about their donor or donor-conceived siblings. Your child may begin calling the donor "the donor" and later call them "the bio dad." They may refer to their donor-related siblings as brothers and sisters. Your child may want to share information about their origins with their friends as they get older, or they may not. Like adults, they may be private people or outgoing. If you're beginning your donor-conception journey, you may feel like you want to cocoon yourself and your partner with your new baby and experience this very intimate and sacred relationship the three of you share without the interference of someone who can feel like a stranger. But when you become a parent, you will feel and own that special role. You will feel secure as a parent and will want to do all you can for your child. And when your child says, "I really want this amazing ice cream I had in school today," you will want to get it for them. You may even stay up into the middle of the night searching for this special ice cream that your child "must have." Similarly, if they say, "Mom, why do I have dimples and you don't?" you will want to help them with that, too.

Speaking Well of Your Donor

You may be looking at the title of this section and thinking, *Okay, I was with you until this. It feels hard enough to get comfortable with telling my child the story of their donor. Why do I need to talk about the donor's nice qualities?*

There are many reasons, but two are primary for most of the parents we see. First, even if your child feels they are nothing like their donor or are not interested in meeting their donor or donor-related siblings, you never know if this will change. It is important that your child knows you are open to them meeting their genetically linked relatives and that you support them in any choice they make. You want to be an ally in their self-discovery. This may be difficult if you are planning to use, or have used, an anonymous donor to conceive, but knowing you support their search will empower your child and further build your bond.

Second, as we have discussed, your child needs to feel good about all parts of who they are, including the parts that are connected to their donor. They may have dimples while you don't, or they may have different color hair or eyes from you. Whatever it is that is different from you, it's good for them to hear that those are qualities you like or admire as much as the qualities that are similar to you. This may be difficult. Even people who are genetically connected to their children like to boast that their daughter is great at math like they were at the same age, for example. It may take a little work to remind yourself to do this, but you don't need to go overboard. Say what you can say genuinely and with a full heart. Maybe you know that your donor had several pets. You could tell your child that she must have a big heart to care for so many animals. Maybe your donor transferred schools so she could play sports. You could tell your child how talented and ambitious she must be. Your child may take these messages to heart, or they may not think much about them. Three children in a family can hear the same message and interpret it totally differently. But at least you put some warm and respectful feelings out there for your child to absorb.

Speaking well of your donor can also help protect them from hurt. A few years ago, I (Mark) noticed that my son, who was five at the time, seemed to be withdrawn and looking inward. After this went on for a week or so, I asked him about it. He told me that some kids on the kindergarten playground had told him he must have a mom, and he must be adopted. This comment not only pointed out to him that his family is different, but it also led to his believing that he had been "given away" (the children's words) by somebody else. This was a heartbreaking moment, but also a teachable one.

Our son had always been told that there is a special woman who gave us some special cells that were combined with Daddy's and Papa's to make him. Though he knew this story, at the age of five, he didn't have the tools to fully understand how he came to our family. What he did understand was that this woman was indeed special—he'd always heard kind, positive things about her. So, when I spoke to him—kindly, but also very directly—about what he'd heard at school, I reminded him about that special person. I told him that not only did nobody give him away, but he is one of the most treasured, wanted children on the planet because his parents used every tool in their scientific toolbox to bring him to life. While many mommies and daddies have babies, they don't meet their children until they're born, and we got to meet him as a tiny little ball of cells before he was even placed inside his surrogate's utcrus. And it was at that point in time that we began to love him. And want him. And we could not have done it without that special woman.

My (Lisa's) children have known from day one about their birth parents. They knew they were placed with us with loving hearts. In adoption, this is not always easy to navigate. My children also know that some people grow in their mommy's tummy and some children grow in "other ladies' tummies." Since all three of my children have very different stories and genetic backgrounds, their experiences learning about their stories have never been straightforward. They have also never been straightforward because all children are different and digest information differently. All children have different personalities and may have different experiences of their birth stories and their birth order in their family. The process of children learning about their beginnings is multifaceted. Remember that no parent is perfect, and we all make mistakes. One of the most important things you can do is be consistently loving and consistently respectful and thoughtful about your donor.

Concerns About Privacy

Some people worry that if they tell their child their donor-conception story, they will share it with others, like at school. We understand this concern but do not see it happen often. Young children are typically more concerned about what will happen on the playground during recess or who they will sit next to in the lunchroom. However, it is a possibility.

As we have said, children don't often grasp the meaning of the story when they are very young. We know one woman who used fertility treatment and was unsuccessful. She then separated from her partner and decided to use donor sperm to have a child as a single mother. She saved for some time to afford treatment, and by then, her eggs had gotten older and she needed an egg donor as well. When she conveyed this story to her son, she told the story in phases, and with each phase, she talked about how she was so excited to have him that she worked hard to save the money and then found a way. When that plan didn't work, she saved money again and found another way, and so on, until she finally found a way to help him come into the world. This little kindergartener knows all about his story, and he doesn't talk about it much, but he did mention to his friends that his mom really wanted him and he was very expensive. His friends nodded, perhaps one said, "Oh, cool," and they continued playing their game.

In this woman's story, as in Mark's story, we see that there are more questions to answer than there are in an opposite-sex family. The degree to which you live in a diverse community is the degree to which this could be challenging. If your child is donor-conceived but you live among many families who "look different," things will likely be less complicated for your children because "everyone" will have a different story. However, if you live in a more homogeneous neighborhood, helping your child field questions about their origins will be even more important. I (Lisa) run workshops for donor-conceived children to help them with this process. Many factors, including their relationships with peers and teachers, will influence how children feel about their story at any particular time in their lives and whether they will or won't disclose to others. Ultimately it will be their decision and their story to share or not to share.

If you have gotten this far in the chapter, congratulations! This is not easy. Much of this may run contrary to all your instincts and trigger your fears. The most important thing you can do now is digest this information—there's a lot here. But the main point is simple: disclosure to your child is critical to their understanding of who they are and how they came into this world. Understanding their donor-conception story can help them make sense out of many things. Some of those things are concrete, like why they have freckles or musical talent when nobody else in the family does, and other things may be more vague, like just wanting to know about donor-related siblings. One of the most important jobs for every parent is to help their children feel good about who they are.

The Importance of Listening

This brings us to our last point in this chapter. Whether you have a strong desire or are reluctant to disclose to your child, it's important that you do not project onto them your feelings of anxiety or sadness. Listen to your child, and explore with them what they need and who they are. Here is one story to illustrate this point.

ALISON

Alison was a single mom who read to her daughter, Audrey, every night before bed. As Audrey moved from kindergarten to first grade, her reading skills increased, and Alison noticed that she was reading more and more by herself. Though Alison loved reading with her daughter, she saw that Audrey loved reading on her own, so she decided to let her read by herself at night. After a couple of weeks of this, Audrey asked her mother a question at bedtime: "Mom, can I meet my donor?"

Inside, Alison panicked. She wondered what to do, what to say, and how she could help her child. Her instinct was to say yes immediately, find her daughter's donor, set up a meeting, and develop a relationship right away. She worried that Audrey was desperate to meet the donor immediately, and she deeply wanted to make Audrey happy and satisfy her curiosity. At the same time, Alison also wondered about Audrey's donor—what she looked like, what it would be like to meet her, and if she would be like Audrey in any way. But Alison's fear of not doing the right thing and her curiosity about Audrey's donor were her own feelings, not Audrey's, as she was about to discover.

Alison took a breath and stayed calm. She tucked a lock of Audrey's wavy dark hair behind her ear and said, "Sure, we can. Are you thinking about your donor?"

"Yes," Audrey said.

"What do you think she would be like?" Alison replied.

"She would be nice," Audrey said.

"I think so, too," Alison said. "In what way do you think she would be nice?"

Audrey said, "I think she would read to me a lot."

"Oh," Alison said, the gears in her mind turning. She said, "Sure, sweetheart, we can meet her." She continued, "I'm wondering, Audrey—are you upset that I don't read to you as much anymore?"

Audrey nodded. "I miss it," she said.

After some discussion, it became clear to Alison that this was what Audrey wanted. At that moment, she did not want to meet her donor. She may in the future, and Alison is ready to help her. But at that moment, she transferred her desires for her mom to read to her more onto her donor. If Alison had just acted on Audrey's first statement without exploring more deeply, she could have missed important information about how Audrey was feeling.

Sometimes feelings about your child's donor are really about your child's donor. And sometimes they may not be. Be sure to listen to your child and remember that what you are feeling may not be the same as what they are feeling. If you take the time to explore with your child at bedtime, in the car, when you're playing a game, you may learn more about your child than you knew.

If disclosing to your child is a struggle and continues to be a struggle, it's helpful to work with a qualified mental health counselor. Earlier, we talked about the fact that you may have two sources of upset when you begin your fertility journey: You may be upset about not having a child and also about not being able to have a fully genetically connected child. Once you have your child, half of that pain is gone. You are a parent and can enjoy so many of the wonders and joys that parenting brings. But it will not change the fact that you used donor conception to build your family, and to be present for your child, embrace their donor (and your child by extension), and work on sharing your child's story with them, you may need to grieve over the losses you have experienced. But remember that issues like your infertility or lack of genetic connection are your issues, and yours to work out. They do not belong to the child. Your child needs you to understand their complex set of feelings, which will be different from yours.

10

Chronicling Your Journey and Building Your Story

After reading the last chapter, you may be feeling relieved that you have a plan for disclosing, or you may be anxious. It may still feel difficult to wrap your head around it. Depending on where you are, you may or may not be ready to take a deeper dive into chronicling and building your story. If you're not ready, that's fine. Put the book down, take a breath, and get back to it a little later. We do recommend you start working on your donor-conception story before or while you're in treatment for many reasons that we'll discuss in this chapter. But first, let's talk about what that story could entail.

Three Elements to Include in Your Narrative

After many years of working with families built with the assistance of donor conception, we have found that an effective narrative includes three main elements: a discussion to explain and develop a tolerance for difference, a discussion about the mechanics of conception and how all people are the same, and your child's own personal story.

Difference

Because your family may look different from the family next door, it's important for children to have a tolerance for difference in general and, by extension, a tolerance for difference in themselves and in their families.

An easy way to start this is through the books you read with your child. There are some great children's books out there on the different ways families are built, such as Todd Parr's *The Family Book*. You can find an extensive book list on the website for the Center for Family Building at www.familybuilding.net, or you can search for your own. The ideas in these books are basically the same. They explain that some families have one dad, some have two moms, some live in an apartment, some live in a house. Some children grow in their mommy's tummy, and some grow in someone else's tummy. All families are beautiful the way they are. What's important to all families is love.

Sameness

Children also need to feel like they fit in. Even the girl in class with the beautiful long red hair will not want to have that beautiful long red hair if it makes her different from her friends. One way to help kids feel like they are the same as their peers is to show them that all people come into the world in the same way. Donor or not, everyone needs a sperm, an egg, and a uterus to come to be. As you begin to bring in more details about egg or sperm donation, not only will your children learn about donor conception but they will also have this idea of sameness reinforced.

On this topic, too, you can find great children's books, like *The Pea That Was Me* by Kim Kluger-Bell. That story shares the basics of how a sperm and an egg go together. There are also books that talk about donor conception in metaphor or in story form. Some of our favorites are included in the list on the Center for Family Building website, but you can find many options through an internet search or by asking a librarian for help. Find a book or style of book that speaks to you and your partner if you have one.

Unfortunately, our society has not yet had a single-parent family in the White House or other prominent position, and while recent years have seen an increase in queer superheroes in the movies and on TV, these figures are still rare. The overwhelming majority of role models children see in our society continue to fit into a small, heteronormative box. Since society doesn't provide many examples of people who look like your family, you can help to create a normative experience for your child yourself. If you can, participate in donor-conception groups or activities. If you're a single parent, try to socialize a bit with another single parent, and if you're a gay or trans parent, try to connect with other LGBTQIA+ families. Seeing these connections can be very helpful for your children.

Living in a cosmopolitan area helps. When I (Lisa) was little, I went to school with kids who had two moms. My parents had gay friends, and so did I. But that was in Greenwich Village in New York in the 1970s. Not everyone has that advantage, so it may be up to you to deliberately find connections for your children. You will help them understand acceptance for the world and for themselves by connecting with others who share similar stories. The Family Equality Council offers programming for LGBTQIA+ families and a wonderful weeklong getaway in Provincetown, Massachusetts. Gay Parents to Be has a library of great information that you can access at https://www.gayparentstobe.com/resource-center. *The Queer Family Podcast* (and its associated book, *If These Ovaries Could Talk*) provides listeners with a wide range of experiences and strategies on LGBTQIA+ family building. And there are more resources for single parents every day. As donor conception continues to become more common, you'll likely find more resources and more opportunities to create these connections.

Your Child's Story

The third part of your narrative is your child's personal story. There are many books that talk about how sperm or egg donation works, and helping your child understand the mechanics of the process is important, but children like to have a story of their own, too. How did your child come into this world? To chronicle that journey for your child, we recommend making a lifebook.

Making a Lifebook

Lifebooks are similar to the classic baby books you may be familiar with, with prompts and spaces for filling in information about all the phases of the journey that led to your child's birth, but this is not about your child's first birthday or first tooth. A lifebook captures the time and culture when your child was imagined. To borrow a phrase from the adoption world, this is the story about how your child began in your heart and came into your home.

Building a Narrative All Your Own

A lifebook doesn't have to be perfect or beautiful, and you don't even have to complete it right now. But it is ideal to start on it while you are beginning your journey. You can write about your surrogate, if you're using one, and about things that you may otherwise forget, like where you went for lunch the first day you met your doctor. What were the thoughts you had and the wishes you held for your future family? What were the funny stories you can share that happened during the pregnancy? As much as it may feel now like these memories will last forever, you will be surprised how much help a lifebook can be in bringing back those moments and details when you want to share them with your child.

Things to record in the lifebook include a letter to your child. You can talk about how you and your partner met, if you have one, and how you felt when discussing your future as parents. It could be helpful to add the reactions of other people and how excited they were for you when you told them you were going to have a child. Be sure to write about things you got excited about, such as things you like about your donor, having a child who will be similar in age to your brother's children, or what your plans for the delivery would be. You can also begin building a family tree. The tree roots would include you and the donor, and the surrogate, if you have one, and the tree leaves would include your entire family. Creating this visual can be very helpful for your child because it provides a visual representation of how they came into the world, who their family is, and all the people who helped. Some may be the same, and some may be different, but the child can see that all these people are connected to them.

We talked in the last chapter about speaking positively about your donor. Well, here's a great place to start. You'll obviously want to include basic information about your donor, but it will also be nice for your child to see you saying nice things about the donor in print. You may do that in person when you disclose to them, but putting those warm comments down on paper can be impactful and reinforce your good feelings for your donor, which will of course translate into good feelings for your child and the way they were created.

I (Lisa) developed *My Lifebook* to help parents-to-be complete a story that is meaningful to them. As children grow, they understand more complicated concepts. *My Lifebook* is grounded in psychology and will help you create your own personal narrative and include information that your child is likely to want to understand. The information will grow with them over time as more complex prompts are included. You can buy a copy through the Center for Family Building website, familybuilding.net, or on Amazon.

My Lifebook is filled with prompts to help you record important information, but you can also create your own lifebook. There's no right or wrong way to do this, but if you're starting from scratch, you'll want to include all the elements discussed above, from the letter to your child to the family tree to a description of the donor. Beyond that, think about things that you want to share with your child. What are your hopes and dreams for your family? Write about that. Write about all the heartfelt experiences, conversations, and ideas you had about your future family before your baby was born. Put yourself in your children's shoes and think about what they might want to know. If you're at a loss, take a look at some of the websites where donor-conceived people write about their desires. The Donor Sibling Registry is also a great place to begin.

Whether you buy *My Lifebook* or make one of your own,

make it personal to your story. Make it fun, and make it yours. In the lifebook I (Lisa) made for my children, I included a story about how my mother used to make me heart-shaped pancakes, and I was looking forward to doing the same for them. I even included a picture of the very imperfect but filled-with-love pancakes.

For the reasons mentioned earlier, it's great to start your lifebook while going through treatment. But if you're not ready to start a lifebook now, just start keeping mementos like your doctor's business card, boarding passes from the trip you took to visit your surrogate, or receipts from the restaurant you went to after the first time you met with your doctor. Store them in a box and write notes in a notebook you can convert to your lifebook later. At the same time, it's never too late to start a lifebook. If you're already a parent, you can still start it now. In my children's workshops, I (Lisa) find that kids love to look at their lifebooks no matter how detailed (or not) they are. Many families also like to work on their book with their child. The child can contribute and become part of the process of creating a book about their story that is special to them.

They don't have to be perfect. I (Lisa) have to admit my lifebooks are a bit of a mess. My family-building story was stressful, and I didn't have the time or presence of mind to make a work of art. But I realized that's okay. The information is there, albeit imperfect, and my kids don't care.

USE TECHNOLOGY

I (Mark) have to admit that in my family, we have not done a wonderful job of creating lifebooks for our kids, and I feel badly about that because I know they would benefit from it. They are now eight and ten, and my husband and I are trying to pull together stories of what happened while we were preparing to get pregnant, while we were pregnant, and who their donor was in the early days surrounding their birth. To collect these, I've set up an email account for this purpose. This is an account my children don't know about yet, but I am constantly emailing them stories, notes, and pictures that we can build into a lifebook later. If you're feeling overwhelmed now and unable to pull together a lifebook, this email hack can be an easy way to get started now. You could also set up a cloud-based folder or blog for the same purpose. What's important is that it's quick and easy to use. I'm often on email, so being able to shoot off a note without changing apps works well for me. Every person needs to find their own way to record the story of how their child came into being.

The lifebook concept has been very popular in the adoption world for decades, but it's not yet as prevalent in the world of donor conception. And many of the books out there are very heteronormative. You are creating a family in an alternate way, and there should be a place for everyone. Ideally, your child will consider you their ally in their self-discovery. Creating a lifebook is one more avenue where your child can connect with you, ask questions, and explore their origins.

Other Benefits to a Lifebook

In addition to helping your child's social-emotional development, a lifebook provides other benefits. As we've discussed in other parts of this book, you can't predict how your child's donor will react if your child reaches out to them at some point. Even if your donor has agreed to connect with them, they may change their mind—particularly if they have had many offspring reaching out to them. It will be important to help your child understand this as they get older and if they want to search. While there is no substitute for meeting their donor, if your child decides one day that is what they want to do, a lifebook that includes information about your donor and the process you went through to create them can help fill in some gaps for your child.

This idea of building a narrative for your child now can be taken further. We have worked with people who have made a video series with their donor for their future child. One couple in particular met with their donor and invited them to their home for the weekend. They took walks, went for bike rides, and had meals together. They felt that the natural flow of conversation would help more information emerge easily and wanted to create a film of these interactions for

236 • LISA SCHUMAN and MARK LEONDIRES

their future child. She was not interested in an ongoing relationship but was willing to share this weekend together. Perhaps they will reunite in the future. For now, they have this beautiful home movie they will probably rewatch again and again with their children.

Another benefit to making a lifebook will affect you more directly and immediately. The donor-conception process can be an anxious time. Choosing a clinic, a donor, an agency, a sperm bank, and a surrogate are all time-consuming processes. Once the pregnancy is stable, however, many people find themselves wishing they still had weekly doctor visits or appointments with multiple professionals to attend. We recommend that you be proactive about addressing your stress and anxiety, and we offer strategies for doing so in chapter 11. In the meantime, it may be helpful to know that chronicling your child's story can also provide you with a valuable activity that can help you feel that there is something within your control, especially when so much of this process can feel out of your control. It can help you feel productive and creative, and ultimately, it will be a great gift to your future child.

Sharing Your Narrative Outside Your Family

Since we're peering into the future at life with a donor-conceived child, what does that life look like, anyway? Well, most days you will be busy changing diapers and just getting through life on little sleep. The baby fog is real! Then, as your children grow, you will be busy with soccer practice or swim lessons, and you will become accustomed to sharing your life with this little person who means the world to you. In other words, you will acclimate to parenthood. While it's unlikely you'll ever look back on these days of fertility treatment and say, "Oh, that wasn't so bad," the challenges of this time will fade into the background of your life. You will be morphing into the beautiful new version of yourself we call *parent*.

Then, once in a while, something will happen that snaps you back. You may be at the playground with your child or at school pickup, and someone may say, "Hey, your son is such a good athlete / has such natural musical talent / is so good at math for his age. Which one of you does that come from?" In that moment, you will remember your donor's contribution to your son's talent. You may feel good that your child did not inherit your two left feet or perhaps feel sad that someone else's genetics were needed to create your family. Other times, you may encounter intrusive questions and tone-deaf comments, such as "Where is little Sammy's mom/dad?" "Who is the real dad?" or "It's amazing how much your child looks like you, and she's not even yours." These comments often come from a place of curiosity and are not intended to hurt, but nevertheless they can hurt.

Families who use donor conception to have their children need to decide how to manage these comments from the outside world. It can be difficult. You may experience a lot of hurt feelings before you become comfortable with your go-to responses. You may also regret sharing too much, because once it's out, you can't take it back. Say you're standing outside the preschool waiting for the kids to get out, and your guard is down, and you share a bit more than you mean to about your donor with a fellow mom. That person may be a Chatty Cathy who goes on to share those things with other parents or others in the community—things that were personal and precious to you.

Perhaps you shared your plans to use a donor with friends with whom you felt close—maybe the fertility treatment felt monumental and you wanted to share your angst, or you wanted to share your joy in choosing your donor. Maybe you love the idea of openness and have wanted to be open with family and friends from the very beginning. These scenarios are natural, and while you are going through treatment, your circle may be small. You may have a close group of friends and family members who are in your corner and have helped you along the way. But soon you will be in the baby music class, then the play group, then preschool, Girl Scouts, and soccer practice. Your network will widen, and continue to widen, and the people in your world may have questions—perhaps personal, sometimes nosy, maybe even invasive. Managing such questions and deciding what to share in those moments can be a very different experience from sharing with those people you are closer with. That's why now is the time to start thoughtfully considering how you will handle your story with others so you'll be ready when the mom from ballet class starts to quiz you.

This may seem controversial, especially considering that

we are so open about this topic and believe in transparency in most things in life, but here we go: We truly believe that no matter how open you want to be, if you believe someone is not going to be supportive of your decision to use donor conception to have a child, don't tell them—or tell them as little as possible. This goes for family members and friends as well as that random parent at the playground.

For example, I (Lisa) shared some of my children's birth family information with one of the aides in my daughter's school. She was an immigrant and raised in a very religious culture. She came from a patriarchal society and didn't understand why someone would be a parent if God didn't grant parenthood for them. But I really liked her and ignored these red flags, so I told her all about my journey and how my children came into my life. For years, at every school event, she said things like, "Of course this is not for you—your child doesn't come from you, so you don't really understand her." Comments like these continued for the next several years while my daughter attended that school. I tried to educate this woman, but she did not understand. I know she didn't mean to be hurtful, but it did hurt. If I had to do it over again, I would have not shared my children's birth information with her. People have all kinds of ideas about donors, and people may also have negative ideas about your donor. Hearing those things can be hurtful as well—for you *and* your child.

As for me (Mark), my husband and I decided early on that which child is genetically linked to whom would be private in our family. We both agreed that the kids would be the first ones to know, and we have held to that in spite of the occasional nosy questioning from outsiders. Once, when our second child was a year old and I was walking both boys in the double stroller down by the beach, I ran into a woman, a stranger, who stopped and cooed at them. "Are you giving your wife the day off?" she asked. I blithely responded, "No, we are a two-dad family." She paused, acknowledging the statement, and then asked, "Which one is yours?" I was shocked, but prepared, and responded, "They're both mine." To this, she replied, "But which one is *really* yours?" "Well," I said to her, "that is something that's private to our family, and when they want to know, we will share it with them. If you are part of our life then, you can find out then."

This "who's the daddy" business is a reminder of our heteronormative world. I get it, but in our families, parenting has nothing to do with genetics. We believe our children's privacy and their story belongs to them, so unless there is a medical reason to discuss who the "bio-parent" is, it can remain part of a story yet to be told.

Privacy Versus Secrecy

Over time, more research will be done, and we will have more information about donor conception and all the feelings it brings. For now, it's helpful to think about the difference between privacy and secrecy. When some families begin their journey to use donor conception, they can feel shame—shame about what they feel their bodies could not do, shame that they won't "be like everyone else," shame that their parents will be disappointed to learn they will not be grandparents to a genetically related grandchild.

Shame hurts, and shame poisons you and everyone around you. And it may fuel a desire for secrecy.

Privacy, on the other hand, is about respect. Here are some examples. What if your child does not want to share information about their donor with their teacher? Should they? What if your mother-in-law criticizes every choice you make? Do you need to tell her which clinic, donor, or agency you chose? The answer to both is no, you don't. And keeping that information to yourself is not keeping a secret; it's making a reasonable, respectful decision about information that teacher or relative does not need to know.

For many, privacy can feel shameful. Sometimes people believe that if they don't shout every detail of their family-building process from the rooftops, they must be ashamed of the way they built their family. This is simply not true. You can be respectful of everyone involved, honor your child's donor, and still reserve the right to privacy when needed.

Everyone is entitled to be who they are. In my (Lisa's) workshops, I help children understand their story and how to disclose or not disclose to others. One piece of this has to do with their temperament, and this applies to parents, too. Just like your child, you are entitled to be outgoing or private, shy or talkative, serious or comical. These temperaments, mixed with your partner's temperament and your unique story, will combine to create your way of telling or not telling others. Yes, it's important to be proud of the way you built your family, but it's also important to be respectful of your unique personality, your unique circumstances, and the unique personality of your child.

Issues Specific to Single Parents-to-Be and Same-Sex Couples

If you are a single or an LGBTQIA+ parent-to-be, it will be clear to others that you did not get pregnant without assistance. People often want all the details, and your child could feel, as one of my (Lisa's) patients once said, "like an exotic pineapple that everyone wants to look at." It can create an uncomfortable situation. However, you do not need to feel obligated to provide any information to people who ask, such as who is the genetically linked parent or specific information about your donor. When people know who the genetically linked parent is, that can set up expectations about the child's traits that can pigeonhole the child. For example, if the genetically linked parent is very athletic, people may assume the child will be athletic, or teachers may think the genetically linked parent who is an accountant will inevitably pass down their math skills to the child. It can also marginalize the other parent. In these situations, even well-meaning people may not realize that there is another parent who is loving and influencing the child's growth and development every day.

As I (Mark) described above, I have found that "We are a two-dad family" is really effective because it says I am gay, I have a partner, and this is my child—all in one. Sometimes people will press: "No, I mean whose sperm/egg did you use?" When they do, it's helpful to have a response ready. One common dilemma that can be a challenge early on is when someone says, "The baby looks just like you," to one of the parents. When that happens, you can reply, "The baby really looks just like the donor." The inquisitor will not have seen the donor and will be forced to reset what they see.

Many queer individuals have parents who feared their child would not make them a grandparent and are delighted to hear that they will be grandparents after all. This makes everyone feel good, but it also highlights "difference." Things like where you live, your cultural norms, and religious beliefs can influence how your family will feel about your partner and your children. Therefore, your announcement about your plans for family building can bring joy and excitement, or generate anxiety or make others upset.

Families are complex, and one person may want to educate their relatives about their family, or family-to-be, while others decide to create some distance between them and their family members who do not embrace them. There are many ways to approach this, and you should feel empowered to choose the approach that works best for you.

Make a Plan for Sharing—Or Not Sharing

If you're on the fence about talking to friends or family members, you can wait. Many people are unsure if their families will be accepting or not and feel caught between wanting to be open and wanting to be self-protective. If this is you, you can put off disclosing to people with whom you

244 • LISA SCHUMAN and MARK LEONDIRES

are not close. You may want to enjoy parenthood, allow the outside world to know your child for who they are, and decide how much you want to share or not share. You are entitled to make privacy decisions about sharing your child's donor information with others, especially if you know those people will be hurtful to you or your children.

Just like it is important to practice your child's birth story before they understand, it's also helpful to practice responses to friends and family ahead of time. First, speak with your partner, if you have one, about their point of view. You may have to compromise to arrive on a mutually agreeable solution. Yes, compromise. Sometimes neither party can get what they want, but they can develop a mutually agreeable plan that will consider both people's feelings. Talk about all the scenarios you can imagine. What if grandma says something uncomfortable or your best friend wants every detail? How will you manage the questions in the supermarket, the schools, and on playdates? It's healthy for your relationship to be on the same page, and it's immensely useful to arm yourselves with responses before the questions come. Getting caught off guard feels terrible, and you don't want to regret saying something that fell out of your mouth in the heat of the moment.

Family dynamics can be complicated. You may decide not to share that you used a donor, or information about your donor, with your grandfather who would be heartbroken to know that your son is not from the same Irish heritage. On the other hand, you may decide you don't care what Grandpa thinks. You may feel comfortable disclosing that you used a donor but not information about your donor or journey. The choice is yours. Just make sure you work it through together so you can be a united front on the subjects that matter most to you and your family.

11

Managing Stress

Whether you're well into the donor-conception process already or are still on the front end, you're well aware of the emotional toll it can take. But the stress, depression, and anxiety you're likely to experience don't just feel bad. These emotions can affect your health and your ability to manage treatment. It's difficult to think clearly when you feel down or anxious, and all the decisions you need to make along the way are too important to address in haste or without a clear head. Stress can make difficult times feel more difficult, and it can make the many periods of anxious waiting—for example, for test results, appointments, or a surrogate—feel twice as long. The emotional duress of treatment can also affect your relationships. Sometimes patients, especially those who have experienced disappointments in fertility treatment, can become so frustrated they decide they "don't care" if a friendship or relationship with a relative is damaged. But these may be relationships that are important to you, and after treatment is over, you may regret letting them unravel.

That's why managing your stress is so important. Many people drop out of treatment because it's too stressful,[1] so it's worth emphasizing the obvious here: You need to complete treatment to have a child. If you drop out of treatment, you won't be able to achieve your dream. We have found the strategies in this chapter to be effective in helping patients think about ways to stay on course more successfully and minimize the collateral damage of possibly letting their self-care slide and tarnishing relationships along the way.

We're providing an introduction—often just the tip of the iceberg—to most of these treatment options and strategies. As you look through these offerings, take note if something resonates with you and then take a deeper dive into that strategy. You can get a lot more out of these ideas by accessing resources like books, YouTube videos, online classes and tutorials, and local classes. Try lots of ideas, and embrace the ones that work for you more fully.

Don't underestimate the importance of caring for your mind and your body. Billionaire Warren Buffett has said that if people knew they had one car for their entire lives, they would take good care of that car. They would make sure the car had its regular checkups, that the car was cleaned regularly, and all problems were addressed immediately. Yet we often take our health and bodies for granted. We skip workouts, reward ourselves by eating junk food, and don't take the time to do things that can help our bodies function well like reducing stress, eating healthy food, and getting a good night's sleep. Surely our bodies are more important than a car, and proactively and deliberately managing our physical and emotional health has far more benefit to us than taking care of a car.

Before we get to the menu of stress-reduction strategies, let's talk about some of the specific issues that different types of fertility patients experience.

Infertility Patients

As we have discussed, infertility can cause a wide range of emotions, including stress, grief, self-recrimination, depression, anxiety, and fear. It can also cause a rift in the family and in the relationship between the couple.

Here are some of the emotional challenges that infertility patients may face.

Grief and Loss

The losses you may have felt can be numerous. The loss of the dreamed-of child, the loss of what you thought your life would look like, the loss of what you thought you and your partner were going to experience together. Losses need to be grieved so we don't get stuck in the past.

When we grieve, we are moving toward accepting what is, even when it feels uncomfortable. When we accept what is, we leave our bodies more receptive to opportunities in the future. If, on the other hand, we practice the pain of our past by running it over and over in our minds, or worse, by making it part of who we are (have you ever said, "Just my luck," or "Nothing ever works out for me"?), we are creating a habit.

Ruminating about something over which you have little or no control is your mind trying to fix the problem. But many of these problems can't be fixed—you can't go back in time and get pregnant earlier, for example, or just not have premature ovarian failure. In these cases, the rumination can act like a bulldozer, digging a moat deeper and deeper around the castle of your mind. Your brain may continue to feel more and more committed to this problem, the unfairness of it, your anger about it. You spend fruitless hours searching for solutions to the problem online or talking about it with your partner, only to get more and more frustrated. Before you know it, the moat has gotten so deep that the you that you once knew is isolated and difficult to reach.

So, what do you do when the reality of a loss does not sit well with you? When it feels so hurtful that you can hardly stomach it? Remember that grieving is a process, and allow yourself, to the degree that you are able, to accept the process. If it feels unbearable, you may need the assistance of a qualified mental health professional to walk you through it. Many also benefit from medication. What's most important is not to deny it. It's not necessary to feel your feelings every moment of every day, but loss needs to be processed, even if it's a little at a time. Otherwise, it gets stuck and often comes out in other ways.

The first stage of grief is denial, which can be experienced as shock. It may take some time for your body to digest your loss fully. You can use calming strategies, such as meditation, to help absorb the shock (meditation is explored on page 263). Try to remain mindful of any negative or fatalistic self-talk while you grieve, and work deliberately to turn back those thoughts or turn them around (page 269).

There are many strategies to manage loss. One of them is to have a ritual. A ritual can help you close a chapter by helping you honor what you have been through. It can help you and your partner make the next steps feel more real. Sometimes when the next step in family building is difficult to accept, an open and outward action that moves you from the past to the present can feel very powerful. You may want to write a letter to the baby that could not be. You may want to put your old ultrasound pictures and information about your appointments or medication in a box and bury it. You may want to plant a tree in its place. There are many rituals that can feel cathartic. If you have had a pregnancy loss, doing this can feel especially important. Most people don't outwardly acknowledge an early loss, but, like a later loss, they also deserve acknowledgment, care, and an opportunity to be marked with a ritual.

Moving from shock to acceptance can take time. Elisabeth Kübler-Ross created a framework for grieving.[2] The stages of grief—denial, anger, bargaining, depression, and acceptance—are natural and can be expected. But sometimes one stage is skipped over, or you may return to an earlier stage again. You need to accept your own process and allow your body and spirit to heal. Does this mean that you can't also take steps forward while you are mourning? We don't mean to suggest that at all. No growth is linear, and it is very common to have feelings of loss or grief resurface years after you have built your family. That is okay. You can have your moments of sadness about what you lost and at the same time be very happy and grateful for what you have. Giving yourself the room to mourn honors your hopes, wishes, and dreams, and can help you commit to your future.

Depressive or Anxious Feelings

If you find that you are not able to perform basic tasks or are excessively eating, drinking alcohol, or doing other self-destructive things to manage your feelings of depression or anxiety, it's important to seek professional help. And if you are having suicidal or homicidal thoughts, please talk to your doctor or go to the nearest emergency room. People resist doing these things because they're afraid for others to see them—or for them to see themselves—as "crazy." Some people, even those who manage their lives very well, have hit very low emotional states when going through fertility treatment. There is no shame in getting help. You must care for yourself if you want to move forward to build a family.

Your experience through fertility treatment is not the only thing that can cause you to become anxious or depressed. Negative self-talk is arguably the most lethal poison to your system and is, unfortunately, common when fertility treatment is unsuccessful, especially for women. If you allow negative self-talk to invade your psyche, it can increase your feelings of depression or anxiety and slow down the acceptance process. Managing negative self-talk can take some work, especially for those who have been doing it most of their lives. But there are many strategies available to help you, and if you're able to get negative self-talk under control, it can make a world of difference in your life.

Concerns About Legitimacy

Many people feel that having a donor-conceived child means they are not the legitimate parent of that child. People who have experienced infertility sometimes feel they don't have the "right" to have a child or fear they will not feel like the child's parent.

It can be difficult to imagine what it will be like to be a parent, and sometimes—after all the disappointments and heartache—it can be difficult to feel *entitled* to become a parent. For many women, having a child seems like a rite of passage, and they believe if they are not getting pregnant, then they have failed, their bodies have failed them, or in some way they are defective. Some women even believe they are different from others who get pregnant easily, and therefore they are not entitled to parent like others.

While it is not easy, it's essential to remember that if parenting is more important to you than having a genetically related child, you can parent. The fact that it is not easy, or that your reality does not match your expectation or your dream, does not mean that you are less entitled to become a parent than anyone else. When you hold that baby in your arms, care for that baby, and share that baby with all the people in your world, there will be no question that your baby is yours. Yes, it will be different, and yes, the donor is now part of your story and your child's story, but you can still enjoy all the great things parenting brings. If you continue to feel like you are not entitled to parent a child, we urge you to seek counseling with a qualified professional to work through the issues that hold you back. In my (Lisa's) more than two decades of working with thousands of fertility patients, I rarely see someone continue to struggle with nongenetic parenthood. Postpartum depression and other emotional difficulties are real and should be taken seriously, but good help is available, so if you need it, don't hesitate to get it. It can make a world of difference in your life.

LGBTQIA+ Patients

There is no one right path for anyone for family building. Perhaps you have experienced this in your coming-out process. For some, it's relatively easy, and for others, it can be heartbreaking. This section briefly describes some of the struggles we have seen LGBTQIA+ patients face, from the most basic to the most difficult. Our hope is that no matter where you see yourself, you will be reminded that you are not alone. Many have come before you and triumphed over these hurdles and are enjoying their families fully. Fertility treatment can be a grueling process necessitating money, time, energy, and patience, but when it's not an option to get pregnant at home, like a straight couple, adoption and fertility treatment are your choices. We have confidence we will see the day when same-sex couples can put together their genetics and have a baby, but we're not there yet. Until then, if you choose donor conception as a way to help build your family, you're likely to need plenty of support, lots of resources, and many of the stress-reduction techniques listed below. But success is possible, and we have your back!

Learning About the Birds and the Bees

Straight couples may get pregnant at home and never think about how it all happened, but for same-sex couples, conception is something they need to learn about and approach deliberately. Conception may happen with insemination or outside the body with the help of fertility professionals, and for some, initiating this process feels intimidating even before they begin. Research shows there is a lot of distrust of the medical profession within the queer community under any circumstances, to say nothing of a circumstance that is so personal and sensitive as family building.[3] Now you need to trust that your doctor will not only be respectful and knowledgeable but that they will also shepherd you along the family-building journey with clarity, kindness, and warmth. You need to trust they know what they're doing and will help you achieve your goal of having a healthy baby. What you need, in sum, is a practice that is both queer-friendly and has good success rates. You don't need to sacrifice one for the other, yet many people do. They are so grateful to have a queer-friendly doctor that they don't consider success rates. Fortunately, this is changing, and more queer couples feel confident and empowered to ask for both.

Once you start your process, there is so much to learn about eggs and sperm, hormones and procedures, it can be mind-boggling. Then there is the legal paperwork and decisions to be made about your donor, openness, who will carry, and where you will find a surrogate or an agency. You will need more of all these procedures and legal documents than many straight couples. On top of that, so much of family building is still unregulated, so make sure you get solid advice every step of the way. It will help the process go more smoothly, calm your anxiety, and help you avoid regrets. If you're feeling insecure about your right to build the family of your dreams, this process may prove to be even more challenging. Thankfully, qualified mental health professionals who have worked with queer couples for decades can help. Be sure to lean on them.

Since there is so much to do, some patients feel an urge to get through it quickly, but it is in your best interest to think through each step and continue to ask questions. We've addressed how important it is to be educated about choosing a donor and the benefits of openness, but even in the treatment process, there are many steps along the way where a little extra attention can be valuable. For example, if you're a gay male couple, consider being present for the embryo transfer to your gestational carrier. This can be a beautiful experience and can help you feel like you are beginning the conception process in a very real way. For lesbian couples, consider how you will both be celebrated, as the person who is not carrying may feel left out at the doctor appointments, baby shower, or even in discussions about the pregnancy with family and friends.

Insecurities can crop up even after the baby is born. I (Lisa) cannot count how many new gay dads have asked me for baby tips. I often remind them that women are in the same boat. No baby comes with an instruction manual. Yet because they are two men, they think they will automatically know less.

Worries About the Children

Research shows that gay families are doing well.[4] Gay families are in the media every day. Yet some queer parents continue to have fears—fears that they won't be good parents, or fears that the children will resent them for not having a different-sex parent or for using donor conception. Gay parents also worry about whether friends and family and the wider world will accept them.

You may have general fears—for example, about traveling to unfriendly countries or states. You may have specific fears, like how your aunt Sarah, who could never accept your boyfriend as your boyfriend, is going to react to the pregnancy. Or you may have fears that are informed by your previous experiences, such as the other families in your child's school treating you the same way you were treated in middle school, or your pediatrician looking at you the way your very religious sister looks at you at family gatherings.

There is an expression that you should trust God but

don't forget to lock your car. The same logic applies here. The truth is that there are many places gay families can live and feel safe, but it is important to have your legal paperwork in place just in case. There are still incidents where families do not cross all their t's and have difficulty making medical decisions for their child who is not genetically related or may struggle to be seen as equal in some courts in a separation agreement. So do all you need to do to reduce excess stress so you can enjoy the process. That may mean getting a second parent adoption and having your wills and power of attorney in place. For some queer couples who are not married, it may be helpful to consider that, too. Political and cultural shifts can make us all feel like the rug is getting pulled out from underneath us at any time. Having all the protections available to you in place can be a very helpful move for you and your family.

Single Parents

Similar to the feelings of infertile women, single parents-to-be can have feelings of unworthiness. However, single parents are also faced with the difficulty of bucking the norm. These feelings of unworthiness, difference, or "selfishness" for pursuing single parenthood can be toxic.

The research on single parents is not clear, but that's because many of the single-parent families that have been studied include divorced households where struggle and strife can be the norm. Many of the single parents we see at the clinic, and many of the Single Mothers by Choice I (Lisa) have worked with or observed, have happy families. That does not mean it's easy to do, but it can be done. And while you are doing it, it is essential, as we have said earlier, to receive support. You will function much better and have an easier path to parenthood if your supports are countering those negative internal messages.

A Word About Adoption

Some of these parents-to-be say something along the lines of, "I may as well adopt because there are so many children out there who need a home." Having also worked in the adoption world for decades, I (Lisa) can attest to the fact that adopting is no piece of cake. First, international adoption has become much more difficult over the past decades. Second, drug use has increased in the United States, which means more babies available for adoption are exposed to drugs in utero. As a result of the narrowing options for adopting a healthy baby and the increasing competition to adopt a healthy baby, adoption has become more intense.

Since there is so much competition for healthy babies, it's unlikely that one of those healthy newborn babies will not be adopted. On the other hand, there are many children in the foster care system with special needs who do not have a home and need one. There are many special people in this world who are willing to adopt or foster children who have special needs, and for many, adoption is a wonderful option. However, it does necessitate a greater leap of faith. Birth mothers do not typically undergo psychological or genetic screening, and it is not common to have full medical records from the beginning of the pregnancy (when development is so critical). Furthermore, you may not have any information on the genetic father of this child. Some people, when faced with a choice between donor conception and adoption, can only imagine adopting, and if that's you, then you should embrace it. But it's important to know that it is not an easy solution to building your family, and there are typically many more unknowns.

Over the past few decades, success rates in reproductive technology have increased, as have the number of fertility programs available, the number of options for financing, and the public's understanding of fertility treatment. With psychological, medical, and genetic testing all being part of the donor-screening process, you have a tremendous amount of control over the health of the genetic contribution to your future child, and, if you are carrying the pregnancy, over the in-utero experience.

Stress-Reduction Strategies

It's been said that our mind creates the world we live in. Mindset has been credited for the success of businesspeople, athletes, and heads of state. Changing your mindset can change your life long-term and short-term, and it can bring about a happier and more relaxed state. Using stress-reduction techniques is a powerful way to help you change your mindset.

The goal of these strategies is not to snap your fingers and feel differently about everything. Rather, the goal is to move to a better-feeling state. There is a place for sadness and grief, but it's not healthy for us to stay in that place. Our bodies will always look for problems to fix. It's natural to want to focus on problems, but many problems cannot be easily fixed, and for that reason, it's easy to get stuck in the past or worry about the future. Giving yourself the opportunity to have your feelings does not mean that you need to stop treatment, crawl under the covers, and shut yourself out from the world.

Let's think about this example. Someday in the future, your son is getting ready for school, and he trips and falls in the kitchen. His skinned knee is bleeding, and he looks at you with tears running down his face. Your child is upset about his knee and also feels frightened at the sight of his own injury, and in his young mind, he decides the worst thing in the world has just happened. Although you console him, he tells you that he can't go to school. Do you let him stay home? No, you clean the wound, patch it up with a Band-Aid, and give him a big hug. Then you tell him he will be fine and help him finish getting ready for school. You neither ignore his feelings and simply push him to go to school nor do you spend hours upset with him and let him stay home. He needs time for his feelings but also needs to feel empowered and to learn that he can overcome a small injury. This experience will help him build confidence and also teach him that all his feelings are valuable. Why treat yourself any differently?

You may have heard the well-worn sports axiom that the best defense is a good offense. That statement is true here as well. Although we offer some ideas for dealing with your stressors in the moment—the "defense" part—many of these strategies are aimed at keeping your mind and heart more resilient, or at least better able to bounce back from upset. Surfers know they need to catch a wave early to ride it. If they wait too long, the wave will be too big and can come crashing down on them. The same is true for you and stress. Practicing the strategies that help you keep your stress levels lower will help keep most of the incoming waves manageable. At the same time, becoming familiar with those in-the-moment strategies will help you be a good emotional athlete who can catch those bigger waves before they get too big and be more skilled at riding them.

The following suggestions are broken down into three categories: decreasing negative emotions, increasing positive emotions, and managing overwhelm. Most people are inclined to use these techniques in this order, but we suggest you try them all.

Stress reduction is not a one-size-fits-all activity. Everyone reacts differently to the stress of family building with donor conception in different ways. And at different times in your life, different strategies may be helpful. So instead of looking at these as a menu of offerings, where you might just choose one or two, like an appetizer and a main course, look at them as a buffet. Try one or a few from each of the categories and see how they fit. At another time in your life, try others. The main point is not to give up. Sometimes we hear patients say something like, "I tried this one strategy, and it didn't work," or "I didn't like my therapist, so I gave up on therapy." Unfortunately, many people spend more time finding a pair of shoes they like than a therapist or a stress-reduction strategy that works. Finding a therapist to share your hopes, dreams, and fears with is nearly as hard as finding a partner. Our emotions deserve the same attention (or more) as other problems in our lives, and yet most of us spend very little time exercising our muscles of positive self-talk or practicing strategies to keep our stress manageable. I (Mark) had a mantra that I used on a daily basis during my coming-out process, a time when I felt self-loathing, that helped me change my own frame of mind. These things work.

Decreasing Negative Emotions

Move your body. This is a slam dunk: getting exercise helps manage the stress hormone cortisol and makes you feel good (besides simply being good for your overall physical health). Take a walk or run, do a few push-ups in the living room, try a free yoga or exercise video online, or get more serious by taking a class in dance, Pilates, yoga, self-defense, or something else. The main thing is to get your blood pumping, put those muscles to use, and fire up the endorphins. Being mindful of your body doesn't have to cost money. If you're tired of looking at your computer, play a song, dance around the house, and sing out loud. It's almost impossible to feel down while dancing to your favorite song. In my own life, I (Mark) have more easily been able to make some difficult decisions while exercising or on a long run, when the answer seems to come more organically.

Check your posture. When your posture is poor, you tend to feel worse. Think about how you stand or sit when you are feeling upset compared to when you're happy. This is a "fake it till you make it" strategy and is backed by research.[5] So sit up straight, even when you don't feel like it. A small adjustment in posture can change your attitude.

Take care of your mind. During times of crisis, your mind may be in overdrive. The best way to quiet the mind is meditation. Herbert Benson, MD, author of *The Relaxation Response,* was one of the first clinicians to notice that people in areas of the world where meditation was a daily practice could control their heart rate and blood pressure using their breath. He modified these ancient techniques, which have worked well for millions over decades.

Meditation can be used like vitamins or like a bandage. Meditating each day can, like taking daily vitamins, bring you a better overall benefit in your life. That's how I (Lisa) use it. However, when you're stressed or overwhelmed, a ten- to twenty-minute meditation session can bring your stress down a notch—sort of like putting a bandage on a wound.

If you've never meditated, it may seem intimidating or perhaps a little woo-woo. But its benefits are proven, and it's worth trying a few different approaches to find one that works for you. There are many types of meditation and many meditation apps and YouTube videos that are free or low cost. Many of the most popular meditation apps offer a seven- or ten-day free trial. This makes sense because if you can practice every day, it can have a spillover effect (like with vitamins). Meditation will not just benefit you in the moment, it can help keep your mood in a better place.

If you would like to take it a step further, try it twice a day—once first thing in the morning, and once at bedtime. If at least one of those sessions involves gratitude, even better. This can be something like setting the thermostat in your home. When you wake from a restless sleep or are feeling anxious about facing the next day, meditation can set your temperature for that morning. Then, at the end of the day, after a roller coaster of emotions, you can reset the temperature to have a better night's sleep. Just as a thermostat will calibrate your heating system to the temperature you want regardless of what is happening outside, meditation can calibrate your mood regardless of what's happening in your life. Even if you just get up ten minutes early to listen to a quick meditation and put your headphones in at bedtime and drift off to sleep, it can work. And don't give up! Changing your mind and mood can take time. It took me (Lisa) a very long time before my self-care routine became habitual and began to change my mood at baseline.

Practice yoga. Yoga has been called moving meditation, for good reason. If you have trouble sitting still, yoga may be a way for you to quiet your mind while moving your body.

Yoga videos, apps, and classes are ubiquitous these days. If you haven't done much (or any) yoga, we encourage you to start with a few free videos online. If you're able to attend a group with others, perhaps even get outside, it can add even more benefit. Getting out of the house and feeling a sense of community is always good.

Just like meditation, yoga is called a practice because the more you do it, the better the effect. You don't need to be good at it. Yoga is something that you do regularly, build a habit of, and accept yourself in the process of working on it. It's been said that not practicing yoga or meditation because you are not good at it is like saying you don't want to take a shower because you're too dirty.

Engage in therapy. Therapy can be extremely useful. Having someone to regularly speak with and gain support and insight from—and to feel like someone is always in your corner—can make an enormous difference in your life. Although therapy has become more mainstream, many still feel there needs to be a mental illness to seek help from a qualified counselor. Nothing could be further from the truth. Think of it this way: What in your life has prepared you for a donor-conception pathway? Nothing has, because nothing could. Talking with an experienced therapist can help ease your way through what can be a tough time. Our lives are more complicated now than they've been at any other time in human history. Putting your thoughts and emotions into words and hearing them back and then discussing them with a trained mental health professional is incredibly helpful.

Therapy can not only help you through the process of donor conception, it may even provide insight into your life in ways you've never considered before. We believe it can benefit everyone. Therapy can help you solve immediate problems and manage stress, but it can also help you change. Engaging in a long-term therapy relationship can be like listening to a piece of music. A song contains high notes and low notes and places of quiet. None of them alone feels like anything. But when you put them together, at the end, you will have an experience of that piece of music. Similarly, long-term therapy is a commitment for a larger change and a leap of faith. That said, it's important to find a therapist who understands you and donor conception. Shop around to find a good fit, and let your therapist know exactly what your goals are. There are many types of therapy, and you need to find the right type of therapy and therapist to suit your needs.

Try alternative methods. Tapping (or the emotional freedom technique), acupuncture, or even massage are not always the first strategies people use to manage their stress, but all of these can be very helpful as well.

Go on a news diet. While keeping up with the news is important, the stress that naturally develops from ingesting negativity and fear can have a significant effect on your psyche. One news program or a half hour of reading the news is enough to keep you up to date and protect your state of mind. Since negative messages can be so disruptive to your mood, it's best not to watch the news before you go to bed or if you are feeling an increased level of stress.

Go on a social media diet. We doomscroll. We expose ourselves to political anger and hate. We compare ourselves to others. We stress about posting the best, most appealing version of our lives possible. It's no wonder that social media is so closely associated with stress, anxiety, and other negative effects. And when you're trying to build your family, it can feel like everyone out there has babies so easily. But there's an easy solution. A 2018 University of Pennsylvania study found that people felt significantly less anxiety, depression, and loneliness, and had significantly fewer sleep problems when they reduced their social media use to thirty minutes a day.[6] Research shows you can feel the benefits after just one week.

Take turns. If you're in a partnership and have children at home, it's extremely important to give each other time to "take breaks" from the children (and housework). This may mean going to bed earlier so you can get up earlier when the house is quiet, or finding separate activities to do with and without the children.

If you don't have children, take turns with other aspects of your life that are a struggle. And there is no judgment here. Maybe you hate doing the laundry or walking the dog. See if you can take turns with a partner or get some help once in a while. It can feel like a huge relief.

Increase Positive Emotions

Get outside. Moving your body is important, but it's also helpful to take a walk outside when possible. Feeling the sun or wind on your face and smelling the scents outside your home activates your senses and can have a positive effect on your well-being.

Give. When you give to others, you give to yourself. After performing an act of kindness, you may notice that you feel more joy and inner peace. You can donate your time, expertise, or money. You might look for an opportunity in your community—perhaps volunteering in a retirement home or at a school or library, perhaps giving to a community group that is dedicated to an issue that is meaningful to you. There are also many opportunities online, from local to national to international. Causes might benefit the environment, animals, or people. Think about what cause would make you feel good, research it online, and make a difference. Even if it feels a bit effortful, the rewards are numerous.

Laugh. If you're feeling down, burned out, or stressed, a funny movie, book, or video can help pull you out of your slump. Or call up that friend who always cracks you up. Look up your favorite old *SNL* skits or stand-up comics on YouTube. There are many accounts of people finding significant healing through laughter. It's good for your mood and your health.

Connect. Make time to connect with people in and outside of your household. Many religious organizations, community centers, and other groups have online platforms for connecting. Play board games or puzzles with friends. Communication with others is important for everyone.

If you're struggling with family building, it may be a difficult time to connect with certain family members and friends. However, isolation increases negative feelings, so think of ways to connect. You can still set boundaries if you need to. Maybe there are some people you just cannot see because they will say hurtful things or talk about their children all day. But maybe there are some people you can watch a movie with and talk about it afterward. Perhaps you can sign up for a painting class with a friend or relative.

Importantly, if you want to ensure that the family-building topic is off-limits, you can ask for what you need. For example, you may say, "I'd like to make a deal with you. I know you care about me and what I'm going through now. But I'm never sure if I want to talk about it or not. It may depend on the day or what I'm going through at the moment. So how about this? If I want to talk about it, I will bring it up. Otherwise, let's talk about what you made for dinner or which shows you are bingeing." Sometimes this strategy is also very helpful for the other person, who may be wondering if they should bring it up. They may worry that if they don't bring it up, it may show they don't care, but if they do bring it up, they may be too intrusive. This way, they don't have to guess, and you can relax, knowing that an unwanted comment won't be around the corner.

Beyond helping you feel better now, connecting with others can be an investment in your future. One day, you will have a beautiful family, and you likely will want many of those people in your life. There may be certain people who you simply cannot see, even on a limited basis. However, if there are people who you can connect with, without too much discomfort, it may be helpful to keep those connections alive. One day, you may feel glad you did. It can be very helpful to think about who you want in your village, because it will take a village to raise your child.

Think about what you do want more than what

you don't want. As mentioned earlier, our bodies often look for problems to fix, but many of the things that are stressful cannot be fixed, at least not in that moment. You can counteract this reflex by focusing on things you can do rather than things you cannot do. This can take a lot of practice, but even if you can do it part of the time, that is an improvement.

Practice gratitude. The saying "Gratitude will change your attitude" may seem hokey, but it works. Research backs it up. You can start by saying, writing, and thinking about three to five things you are grateful for each day. It's ideal if you can do this in the morning (perhaps with your morning meditation). Or you can put a reminder on your phone or a sticky note on your bathroom mirror, or create a new background on your phone that will remind you to practice gratitude. Your list can include anything from a good cup of coffee to a nice phone call or a good night's sleep. It doesn't need to be large, it just needs to evoke a nice feeling, even a small one.

Managing Overwhelm (Or Feeling Out of Control)

Engage in pleasurable activities that are within your control. This could mean reorganizing your living room, taking an online drawing class, or learning how to knit.

The fight-or-flight response is triggered when the body feels a potential threat is near. Once that fear has passed, the body recovers. For example, if something scares you, your heart may race and the hair may stand up on the back of your neck. When the scary incident is over, the body returns to its natural state. Fertility treatment is full of immediate things that need to be done, changes, and sometimes disappointments. The roller coaster of fertility treatment does not allow time for calm and recovery. Cortisol (the stress hormone) can affect many aspects of your body and increase your feelings of anxiety and sadness. When that happens, you're in the passenger seat and have no control over what's happening. This can be magnified for people in donor conception because your outcome is not only dependent on the clinic and science but also on someone else's body. Not having control over the success or timing of any of these things can feel very dysregulating. Being able to find an activity that is pleasurable (not work-related) can help you feel more in balance. When you put your energy into something pleasurable and see evidence of your efforts, it can feel very grounding. It's great to schedule enjoyable activities, but seeing the results for your efforts is key here. When everything can feel out of control in your world, it can feel very stabilizing to finally see your living room painted, or feel good to complete your plan to hike every trail within a fifty-mile radius of your home by the end of the summer. Starting your lifebook now can be one of those projects. You can create a gift for your future child and have a project that can help tame your anxiety.

If concerns about your finances are part of your experience, you may feel empowered by using some relaxation exercises and then problem solving. Finding new ways to make money and exploring fertility options with your doctor or reproductive therapist are some examples of ways to feel more in control. If this exercise causes more frustration, pursue it for short periods of time or put it on the shelf until you are feeling a greater sense of control.

Stay on a schedule. Going to bed and waking at the same time each day has been shown to be beneficial to your health and emotional well-being. Maintaining your body's typical schedule can help you sleep better at night, help you feel productive, and keep your household in sync.

If you are having a lot of bad luck in your fertility journey or feeling very stressed on your transition to donor conception, it may be worth your while to commit to one or more of the habits described in this chapter. If you feel prepared to start, we suggest focusing on thirty-day increments. The first thirty days can be really difficult. In fact, you may feel like you're walking through quicksand, yanking yourself out of bed early each morning to start that exercise routine or meditation practice. But if you can get through that month, even if it's not perfect—perhaps aim for 20 percent follow-through or better—you may find that your struggle becomes a bit easier. The next thirty days will be less onerous, and the next thirty after that will be even less so. And if you are finding every day extremely challenging, take it one hour at a time, then work your way up to longer periods or sections of your day. Maybe today you just get through the first hour of work remembering to breathe and eat a healthy breakfast. Maybe that's the best you can do, and if so, that's great. It's progress. Smaller goals can be better than big ones because they're typically more achievable. If you push yourself too hard, you may find yourself back at ground zero and feeling upset about "failing." Just as one must when exercising to get stronger physically, we need to build those muscles a little every day.

Managing your stress as you're facing the ups and downs of using donor conception to have a family isn't only about helping you feel better. Stress management can help you maintain your relationships, persevere through challenges and low times, and manage treatment more effectively so you can stay in treatment and achieve your goal of having the family of your dreams.

Part IV

Preparing for Your Family—with Gratitude

12

Love and Intent

We hope this book has helped you on your path to parenthood or even helped you decide that donor conception is not for you. Underlying this is our hope that you feel empowered. You deserve to have children as part of your family if that is your wish. It may not be the family you once dreamed of, but it can be a wonderful family, and that family can bring you joys (and stress) you could have never imagined. The two most important ingredients you will need to begin your journey are love and intent. The information is available and there are many paths to parenthood, and new options, treatments, and discoveries about donor conception and donor-conceived children are happening every day.

As you're likely aware, we're also seeing advances in

attitudes. Stigma about infertility, same-sex families, and single-parent families is fading, even if not as quickly as we would like. So are longstanding heteronormative paradigms, old-fashioned ideas that made women choose between family and career, outdated marriage laws, and myriad prejudices. As these barriers come down, and more people choose donor conception, and more people talk openly about their donor-conception experiences, it will only get easier to build a family this way—easier emotionally, socially, and practically. Unfortunately, at the time of this writing, political shifts are occurring that may create obstacles to advancing science and expanding personal freedoms. However, we are optimistic that the tide will turn again and life for people with families built in alternative ways will continue to become more normalized. As a wise person once said, "We have come too far to have only come this far."

These advances won't only be helpful to future generations. Between the time we write these words and the time you read them, significant positive changes may already have happened. They may be medical advances or updates to research and best practices. Perhaps another celebrity will publicly discuss their choice to use donor conception, raising awareness and acceptance one more notch. Visibility of donor conception is growing week by week, lowering barriers one step at a time. You have allies and resources and some truly mind-boggling science on your side.

To the Donors: Thank You

For this evolving science, for the opportunity it has created to bring more families—and more love—into this world, we are grateful. We've seen the jubilant faces of many new parents, and those faces always give us great joy. We are grateful to the American Society for Reproductive Medicine, which supports education and the advancement of science on an international level for the achievement of parenthood. They are the voice of our industry, and they help make so much of what we do possible. RESOLVE, the national fertility organization in the United States, is also owed an enormous amount of gratitude. They tirelessly educate, advocate for, and support people all over the world, helping them find resources and a sense of belonging they would have never had otherwise. One in eight people in the United States struggles with infertility, and many of those, as well as others who are not infertile, will need donor conception to realize their dream of becoming parents. And to the Family Equality Council, thank you for all your efforts to make family building a more equal playing field.

While family building has changed, biology has not. Single parenthood and LGBTQIA+ family building are now part of the zeitgeist of our society, but it still requires an egg, a sperm, and a uterus. This is great: it levels the playing field and makes everyone's journey into this world equal, which means every type of family, and every member in a family, can understand that we are all created the same way.

But for many—for you, perhaps—it can't happen without a donor, and it's the donors for whom we have the most gratitude of all. And so, on behalf of the millions of families that have been created through donor conception, we want to acknowledge everyone who has donated their gametes. Every single donor went through medical interviews, blood work, and counseling, and is aware that they may have genetically linked children out there they have not met. Donors: Thank you for doing the work. Through your efforts, parents have been born.

As a parent through egg donation who never got to meet their donor, I (Mark) am so thankful for you and your gift that helped bring my family to life.

Hope

As you prospective parents move forward in choosing a donor, faced with thousands of people on a dating app–like web page, flash forward to a moment when you will be talking to your child-to-be, knowing that they will want to know more about this other part of themselves. Think of it as an opportunity for joy in an expanded world as your child learns of and perhaps meets their donor and/or half siblings. Yes, it can be scary right now, but your child does not need to be burdened with your grief or challenges of bringing a child into the world. They will be seeking a better understanding of themselves, and they will gain a broader, more complex understanding of their creation story *and* the world when they consider that somebody else helped their parents become parents.

We want you to walk away from this book with hope. Yes, it's true that not every procedure works, and some people are luckier than others. In spite of the massive progress that's been made in reproductive medicine over the past two decades, it's still not perfect. Even if someone has a 70 percent chance of establishing a healthy pregnancy, there will be people who will fall into that other 30 percent, and that is something we never get used to and that always upsets us. We push ahead and do our best to help those patients have a child and manage the process with the least amount of stress and confusion. And we ask you to approach your journey feeling empowered, educated, and—yes—hopeful, believing that you are going to be a parent, because this is the most successful fertility pathway within any fertility clinic. If you want a child, it may take more determination and grit than you expected, but it will be worth it. Thousands have been there before you, and you are not alone. We have your back.

We also have hope. Someday, everyone who wants to build a family will more easily be able to do so, and we hope that we will see that change happen in our lifetimes. Of more immediate concern, though, is the change that we hope for for you. Our deepest hope is that you, armed with love and intent, go through the most profound transformation we can imagine—the one from patient to parent.

Resources

American Society for Reproductive Medicine
www.asrm.org

Donor Sibling Registry
donorsiblingregistry.com

European Society of Human Reproduction and Embryology
www.eshre.eu

Family Equality
www.familyequality.org

RESOLVE: The National Infertility Association
www.resolve.org

Single Mothers by Choice
www.singlemothersbychoice.org

Human Rights Campaign
www.hrc.org

Lambda Legal
www.lambdalegal.org

References

Andrew, S. "Baby Born from 27-Year-Old Embryo Believed to Have Broken Record Set by Her Big Sister." CNN, December 1, 2020. https://www.cnn.com/2020/12/01/us/baby-frozen-embryo-27-years-trnd/index.html.

Arocho, R., E. B. Lozano, and C. T. Halpern. "Estimates of Donated Sperm Use in the United States: National Survey of Family Growth 1995–2017." *Fertility and Sterility* 112, no. 4 (2019): 718–23. doi: 10.1016/j.fertnstert.2019.05.031.

Carney, D. R., A. J. Cuddy, and A. J. Yap. "Power Posing: Brief Nonverbal Displays Affect Neuroendocrine Levels and Risk Tolerance." *Psychological Science* 21, no. 10 (2010): 1363–8. doi: 10.1177/0956797610383437. Epub 2010 Sep 20. PMID: 20855902.

Centers for Disease Control and Prevention. "Folic Acid Helps Prevent Serious Birth Defects of the Brain and Spine." June 17, 2022. https://www.cdc.gov/ncbddd/folicacid/features/folic-acid-helps-prevent-some-birth-defects.html.

Domar, A. D., A. Broome, P. C. Zuttermeister, M. Seibel, and R. Friedman. "The Prevalence and Predictability of Depression in Infertile Women." *Fertility and Sterility* 58, no. 6 (December 1992): 1158–63. PMID: 1459266.

A. D. Domar, P. C. Zuttermeister, and R. Friedman. "The Psychological Impact of Infertility: A Comparison with Patients with Other Medical Conditions." *Journal of Psychosomatic Obstetrics and Gynaecology* 14, suppl. (1993): 45–52. PMID: 8142988.

Golombok, S. *Modern Families: Parents and Children in New Family Forms.* Cambridge: Cambridge University Press, 2015.

Golombok, S. *We Are Family: The Modern Transformation of Parents and Children.* New York: PublicAffairs, 2020.

Golombok, S., J. Readings, L. Blake, P. Casey, L. Mellish, A. Marks, and V. Jadva. "Children Conceived by Gamete Donation: Psychological Adjustment and Mother-Child Relationships at Age 7." *Journal of Family Psychology* 25, no. 2 (April 2011): 230–9. doi: 10.1037/a0022769. PMID: 21401244; PMCID: PMC3075381.

Greely, H. T. *The End of Sex and the Future of Human Reproduction*. Cambridge, MA: Harvard University Press; reprint edition, 2018.

Gregory, C. "The Five Stages of Grief." Psycom, June 7, 2022. https://www.psycom.net/stages-of-grief.

Harper, J. C., I. Abdul, N. Barnsley, and Y. Ilan-Clarke. "Telling Donor-Conceived Children About Their Conception: Evaluation of the Use of the Donor Conception Network Children's Books." *Reproductive Biomedicine & Society Online* 14 (June 23, 2021): 1–7. doi: 10.1016/j.rbms.2021.06.002. PMID: 34604554; PMCID: PMC8463736.

Human Fertilisation & Embryology Authority. "Trends in Egg and Sperm Donation." 2019. https://www.hfea.gov.uk/media/2808/trends-in-egg-and-sperm-donation-final.pdf.

Hunt, M. G., R. Marx, C. Lipson, and J. Young. "No More FOMO: Limiting Social Media Decreases Loneliness and Depression." *Journal of Social and Clinical Psychology* 37, no. 10 (2018): 751–68

E. Ilioi, L. Blake, V. Jadva, G. Roman, and S. Golombok. "The Role of Age of Disclosure of Biological Origins in the Psychological Wellbeing of Adolescents Conceived by Reproductive Donation: A Longitudinal Study from Age 1 to Age 14." *Journal of Child Psychology and Psychiatry* 58, no. 3 (2017): 315–24. https://doi.org/10.1111/jcpp.12667.

Imrie, S., and S. Golombok. "Long-Term Outcomes of Children Conceived Through Egg Donation and Their Parents: A Review of the Literature." *Fertility and Sterility* 110, no. 7 (December 2018): 1187–93.

Jadva, V., T. Freeman, W. Kramer, and S. Golombok. "The Experiences of Adolescents and Adults Conceived by Sperm Donation: Comparisons by Age of Disclosure and Family Type." *Human Reproduction* 24, no. 8 (2009): 1909–19. doi: 10.1093/humrep/dep110. Epub April 27, 2009. PMID: 19398766.

McGee, G., S. V. Brakman, and A. D. Gurmankin. "Gamete Donation and Anonymity: Disclosure to Children Conceived with Donor Gametes Should Not Be Optional." *Human Reproduction* 16, no. 10 (October 2001): 2033–6. doi: 10.1093/humrep/16.10.2033. PMID: 11574486.

Miller, S. "LGBTQ Families Are on the Cusp of Dramatic Growth, and Millennials Lead the Way." *USA Today,* February 6, 2019. https://www.usatoday

.com/story/news/nation/2019/02/06/lgbtq-millennials-family-building
-parenthood.

Montclair State University. "The Best Time to Disclose Adoption Status to Children." University News blog, July 22, 2019. https://www.montclair.edu
/newscenter/2019/07/22/the-best-time-to-disclose-adoption-status-to-children/.

"Optimizing Natural Fertility: A Committee Opinion." *Fertility and Sterility* 117 (2022): 53–63.

Pasch, L., D. Shehab, S. Gregorich, R. Nachtigall, P. Katz, and N. Adler. "Explaining Differences in How Women and Men Cope with Infertility: Effects of Appraisals." *Fertility and Sterility* 82, suppl. 2 (2004): S102. ISSN 0015–0282. https://doi.org/10.1016/j.fertnstert.2004.07.258.

Perrin, E. C., B. S. Siegel, and the Committee on Psychosocial Aspects of Child and Family Health of the American Academy of Pediatrics. "Promoting the Well-Being of Children Whose Parents Are Gay or Lesbian." *Pediatrics* 131, no. 4 (2013): e1374–83. doi: 10.1542/peds.2013–0377. Epub 2013 Mar 20. PMID: 23519940.

Rooney, K. L., and A. D. Domar. "The Impact of Stress on Fertility Treatment." *Current Opinion in Obstetrics and Gynecology* 28, no. 3 (2016): 198–201. doi: 10.1097/GCO.0000000000000261. PMID: 26907091.

Siegel, D. R., J. Sheeder, W. Kramer, and C. Roeca. "The Age and by Whom a Donor-Conceived Person Receives Information Significantly Effects Their Experience." *Fertility and Sterility* 116, suppl. 3 (2021): E431–32.

Slutsky, J., V. Jadva, T. Freeman, S. Persaud, M. Steele, H. Steele, W. Kramer, and S. Golombok. "Integrating Donor Conception into Identity Development: Adolescents in Fatherless Families." *Fertility and Sterility* 106, no. 1 (2016): 202–8.

Tortelli, B. "The Fear of Discrimination in LGBT Healthcare." Institute for Public Health, Washington University, September 14, 2016. https://publichealth
.wustl.edu/fear-discrimination-lgbt-healthcare/.

University of Manchester. "Family Life After Donor Conception." Economic & Social Research Council. https://hummedia.manchester.ac.uk/schools/soss
/morgancentre/leaflets/Family-Life-After-Donor-Conception_Heterosexual.pdf.

Women & Infants. "Preimplantation Genetic Testing at a Glance." https://
fertility.womenandinfants.org/treatment/preimplantation-genetic-testing.

Wu, K. J. "Scientists Break the Rules of Reproduction by Breeding Mice from Single-Sex Parents." *Smithsonian,* October 12, 2018. https://www.smithsonianmag
.com/science-nature/scientists-break-rules-reproduction-breeding-mice-single
-sex-parents-180970517/.

Notes

Introduction

1. S. Golombok, *We Are Family: The Modern Transformation of Parents and Children* (New York: PublicAffairs, 2020).

2. R. Arocho, E. B. Lozano, and C. T. Halpern, "Estimates of Donated Sperm Use in the United States: National Survey of Family Growth 1995–2017," *Fertility and Sterility* 112, no. 4 (2019): 718–23, doi: 10.1016/j.fertnstert.2019.05.031.

3. Human Fertilisation and Embryology Authority, "Trends in Egg and Sperm Donation," 2019, 1, https://www.hfea.gov.uk/media/2808/trends -in-egg-and-sperm-donation-final.pdf.

4. S. Miller, "LGBTQ Families Are on the Cusp of Dramatic Growth, and Millennials Lead the Way," *USA Today,* February 6, 2019, https://www .usatoday.com/story/news/nation/2019/02/06/lgbtq-millennials-family -building-parenthood.

5. E. Wantman, Society for Assisted Reproductive Technology, personal communication with the authors.

Chapter 1: Accepting Donor Conception

1. A. D. Domar, P. C. Zuttermeister, and R. Friedman, "The Psychological Impact of Infertility: A Comparison with Patients with Other Medical Conditions," *Journal of Psychosomatic Obstetrics & Gynecology* 14, suppl. (1993): 45–52, PMID: 8142988.

2. L. Pasch, D. Shehab, S. Gregorich, R. Nachtigall, P. Katz, and N. Adler, "Explaining Differences in How Women and Men Cope with

Infertility: Effects of Appraisals," *Fertility and Sterility* 82, suppl. 2 (2004): S102, ISSN 0015–0282, https://doi.org/10.1016/j.fertnstert .2004.07.258.

3. A. D. Domar, A. Broome, P. C. Zuttermeister, M. Seibel, and R. Friedman, "The Prevalence and Predictability of Depression in Infertile Women," *Fertility and Sterility* 58, no. 6 (1992): 1158–63, PMID: 1459266.

Chapter 3: Preparing for Pregnancy

1. "Folic Acid: The Best Tool to Prevent Neural Tube Defects," Centers for Disease Control and Prevention, June 17, 2022, https://www.cdc.gov /ncbddd/folicacid/features/folic-acid-helps-prevent-some-birth-defects .html.

2. K. Van Heertum and B. Rossi, "Alcohol and Fertility: How Much Is Too Much?," *Fertility Research and Practice* 3 (July 10, 2017): 10, doi: 10.1186 /s40738-017-0037-x, PMID: 28702207, PMCID: PMC5504800.

Chapter 6: Balancing Practical and Emotional Considerations

1. K. J. Wu, "Scientists Break the Rules of Reproduction by Breeding Mice from Single-Sex Parents," *Smithsonian,* October 12, 2018, https://www .smithsonianmag.com/science-nature/scientists-break-rules-reproduction -breeding-mice-single-sex-parents-180970517/.

Chapter 8: Dealing with Practical and Ethical Dilemmas

1. L. Schuman, S. S. Richlin, R. Mangieri, M. Kelleher, N. Bolger, and M. Leondires, "The Burden of Family Building as a Gay Male Couple: The Majority of Gay Male Couples Seen at a Large Reproductive Medicine Practice Desire a Child with Each of Their Genetics," *Fertility and Sterility* 112, no. 3, suppl. (2019): e60–1.

2. Practice Committee of the Society for Reproductive Endocrinology and Infertility, Quality Assurance Committee of the Society for Assisted Reproductive Technology, and the Practice Committee of the American Society for Reproductive Medicine, "Multiple Gestation Associated with Infertility Therapy: A Committee Opinion," *Fertility and Sterility* 117, no. 3 (2022): 498–511, doi: 10.1016/j.fertnstert.2021.12.016, Epub January 31, 2022, PMID: 35115166.

3. Schuman et al., "The Burden of Family Building as a Gay Male Couple."

4. L. Schuman, S. S. Richlin, M.Kelleher, N. Bolger, and M. P. Leondires "LGBTQ+ Couples and Family Building Priorities: Women Put a Lower Priority on Their Genetics Than Men," *Fertility and Sterility* 118, no. 4, suppl. (2022): e325.

Chapter 9: Disclosure

1. S. Golombok, J. Readings, L. Blake, P. Casey, L. Mellish, A. Marks, and V. Jadva, "Children Conceived by Gamete Donation: Psychological Adjustment and Mother-Child Relationships at Age 7," *Journal of Family Psychology* 25, no. 2 (April 2011): 230–9, doi: 10.1037/a0022769, PMID: 21401244, PMCID: PMC3075381.

2. S. Imrie and S. Golombok, "Long-Term Outcomes of Children Conceived Through Egg Donation and Their Parents: A Review of the Literature," *Fertility and Sterility* 110, no. 7 (December 2018): 1187–93.

3. E. Ilioi, L. Blake, V. Jadva, G. Roman, and S. Golombok, "The Role of Age of Disclosure of Biological Origins in the Psychological Wellbeing of Adolescents Conceived by Reproductive Donation: A Longitudinal Study from Age 1 to Age 14," *Journal of Child Psychology and Psychiatry* 58, no. 3 (2017): 315–24, https://doi.org/10.1111/jcpp.12667.

4. S. Andrew, "Baby Born from 27-Year-Old Embryo Believed to Have Broken Record Set by Her Big Sister," CNN, December 1, 2020, https://www.cnn.com/2020/12/01/us/baby-frozen-embryo-27-years-trnd/index.html.

5. Montclair State University, "The Best Time to Disclose Adoption Status to Children," University News blog, July 22, 2019, https://www.montclair.edu/newscenter/2019/07/22/the-best-time-to-disclose-adoption-status-to-children/.

6. V. Jadva, T. Freeman, W. Kramer, and S. Golombok, "The Experiences of Adolescents and Adults Conceived by Sperm Donation: Comparisons by Age of Disclosure and Family Type," *Human Reproduction* 24, no. 8 (2009): 1909–19, doi: 10.1093/humrep/dep110, Epub April 27, 2009, PMID: 19398766.

7. D. R. Siegel, J. Sheeder, W. Kramer, and C. Roeca, "The Age and by Whom a Donor-Conceived Person Receives Information Significantly Effects Their Experience," *Fertility and Sterility* 116, suppl. 3 (2021): E431–32.

8. J. C. Harper, I. Abdul, N. Barnsley, and Y. Ilan-Clarke, "Telling Donor-Conceived Children About Their Conception: Evaluation of the Use of the Donor Conception Network Children's Books," *Reproductive Biomedicine & Society Online* 14 (June 23, 2021): 1–7, doi: 10.1016/j.rbms.2021.06.002, PMID: 34604554, PMCID: PMC8463736.

9. J. Slutsky, V. Jadva, T. Freeman, S. Persaud, M. Steele, H. Steele, W. Kramer, and S. Golombok, "Integrating Donor Conception into Identity Development: Adolescents in Fatherless Families," *Fertility and Sterility* 106, no. 1 (2016): 202–8.

Chapter 11: Managing Stress

1. K. L. Rooney and A. D. Domar, "The Impact of Stress on Fertility Treatment," *Current Opinion in Obstetrics and Gynecology* 28, no. 3 (2016): 198–201, doi: 10.1097/GCO.0000000000000261, PMID: 26907091.

2. C. Gregory, "The Five Stages of Grief," Psycom, June 7, 2022, https://www.psycom.net/stages-of-grief.

3. B. Tortelli, "The Fear of Discrimination in LGBT Healthcare," Washington University Institute for Public Health, September 14, 2016, https://publichealth.wustl.edu/fear-discrimination-lgbt-healthcare/.

4. E. C. Perrin, B. S. Siegel, and the Committee on Psychosocial Aspects of Child and Family Health of the American Academy of Pediatrics, "Promoting the Well-Being of Children Whose Parents Are Gay or Lesbian," *Pediatrics* 131, no. 4 (2013): e1374–83, doi: 10.1542/peds.2013–0377, Epub March 20, 2013, PMID: 23519940.

5. D. R. Carney, A. J. Cuddy, and A. J. Yap, "Power Posing: Brief Nonverbal Displays Affect Neuroendocrine Levels and Risk Tolerance," *Psychological Science* 21, no. 10 (2010): 1363–8, doi: 10.1177/0956797610383437, Epub September 20, 2010, PMID: 20855902.

6. M. G. Hunt, R. Marx, C. Lipson, and J. Young, "No More FOMO: Limiting Social Media Decreases Loneliness and Depression," *Journal of Social and Clinical Psychology* 37, no. 10 (2018): 751–68.

Acknowledgments

To our amazing agent, Isabelle Bleecker, who believed in us and the immense value in what we had to share. And to our editor, Eileen Rothschild, who had the foresight to know how important this information would be to so many. Thank you.

Index

emotional freedom technique
(tapping), 266
emotions, 4, 164
decreasing negative, 262–70
during embryo transfer, 71–72
egg donors and, 64, 157
health and, 246
increasing positive, 267–70
infertility and, 24–28
managing, 13–14
understanding, 146–49
empowerment, 277
endometrial lining, 70, 95–96
environmental toxins, 98
enzymes, sperm, 48
epigenetics, 78–79, 87, 172–73
equality, marriage, 37
Eric (Amy's partner), 58
estradiol (human estrogen),
62, 75
estrogen, 65, 70
excess embryos, 179–81
exercise, 49, 50, 80–82, 262–63

F

facial recognition, 123
failed cycles, 27
fallopian fluid, 95
fallopian tubes, 49, 91–96
familial donors, 110, 118
family, modern idea of, 44
The Family Book (Parr), 227
family complexity, 243
Family Equality Council,
38, 229, 279
family history, 104, 105
family narrative, 236–45
family support, 2, 196
family traits, 163
family tree, 107, 110, 151
FAS. *See* fetal alcohol syndrome
fate, 33

female child, 151–52
fertility, 7. *See also* infertility
fertility laboratories, 54
fertility treatment, 1, 7, 25,
32, 183
LGBTQIA+ patients and,
253–54
stress management and,
247, 271
fertilization, 46, 48–49, 56,
65–68. *See also* in vitro
fertilization
success rates of, 57
fetal alcohol syndrome (FAS), 86
fetus, 46, 68
fibroid. *See* leiomyomata
finances, 2, 34, 183, 195
stress management and, 271–72
financial reimbursement, 198
fish, mercury and, 98
fluid, fallopian, 95
folic acid, 84–85, 86
follicle, ovarian, 60–63, 76
follicles, 63
follicle-stimulating hormone
(FSH), 61, 74, 75
foster care system, 141, 258
friends, pregnancy and, 27
frozen eggs, 53, 54–57
frozen embryos, 200
FSH. *See* follicle-stimulating
hormone
future-contact agreement, 140

G

gamete donation, 11
Gay Parents to Be (organization),
10, 36, 130–31, 229
gender roles, 193
gender stereotypes, 12
gene expression, 78–79
genetic connection, 28

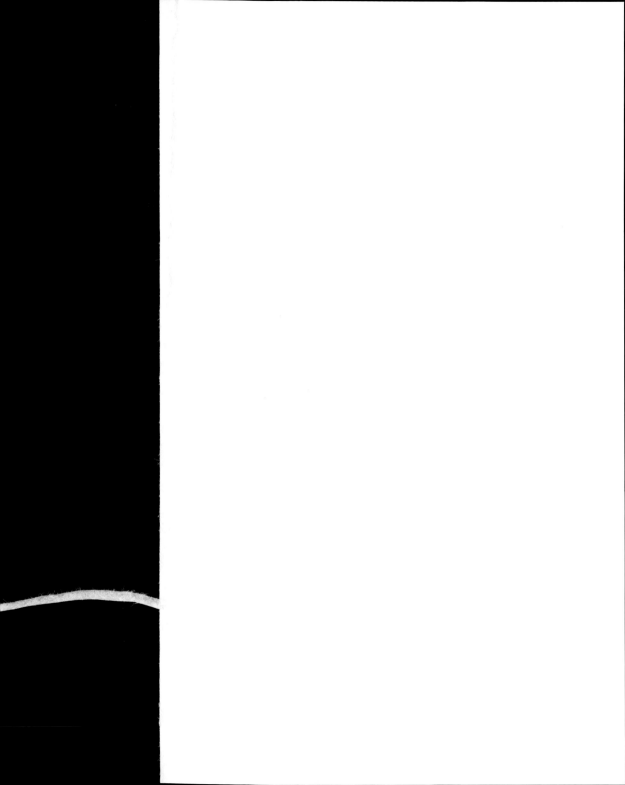

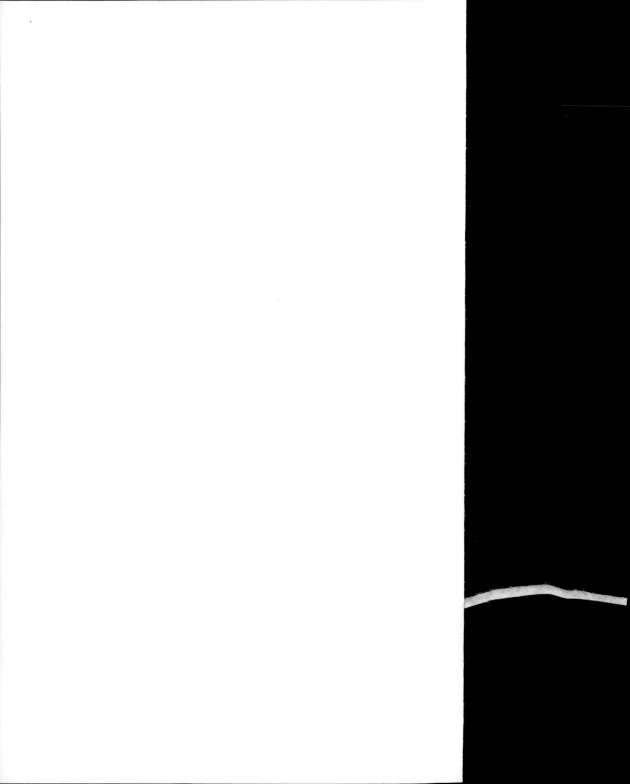